"...The world remains a complex, dynamic, and dangerous place. It will continue to be an uncertain security environment, one for which U.S. Special Operations Forces are uniquely situated, offering the capabilities to avert emerging threats and providing unprecedented opportunities to address the challenges in ways that advance U.S. interests."

— from the Special Operations Posture Statement, 2000

THE SPECIAL OPS WORKOUT

The Elite Exercise Program

Inspired by the

United States

Special Operations Command

by **Mike Mejia & Stewart Smith, USN (SEAL)**

Photographs by Peter Field Peck

A GETFITNOW.COM BOOK

New York

THE SPECIAL OPS WORKOUT:
The Elite Exercise Program Inspired by The United States Special Operations Command

Mike Mejia and Stewart Smith

GetFitNow.com Books / Hatherleigh Press
5-22 46th Avenue, Suite 200
Long Island City, NY 11101
1-800-528-2550
www.getfitnow.com

Neither the specific organizations indicated nor any other component of the Department of Defense have approved or authorized this product. The use of the term "Special Ops" does not express an endorsement, either explicit or implicit, by the United States Military or any of its branches. In all cases, seek the advice of your physician before starting any physical fitness program.

Consult your physician before beginning any exercise program. The author and publisher disclaim any liability, personal or professional, resulting from the application or misapplication of any of the information in this book. The information is provided for entertainment purposes only and is not intended to substitute for proper medical advice and treatment.

Library of Congress Cataloging-in-Publication Data

Smith, Stewart, 1969-
The Special Ops workout : the elite exercise program inspired by the
United States Special Operations Command / by Stewart Smith and Mike
Mejia ; photographed by Peter Field Peck.
     p. cm.
ISBN 978-1-57826-132-1 (pbk. : alk. paper)
1. Exercise. 2. Physical fitness. 3. U.S. Special Operations
Command. I. Mejia, Michael. II. Title.
GV481.S6445 2004
613.7'1--dc22
                                        2003017851

ISBN 978-1-57826-132-1

All GetFitNow.com titles are available for special promotions and premiums. For more information, please call 1-800-528-2550 and ask for the manager of our Special Sales department.

Cover & Interior design by Tai Blanche
Photographs by Peter Field Peck

20 19 18 17 16 15
Printed in the United States of America

CONTENTS

Foreword **7**
by Stew Smith, USN (SEAL)

Part I: Introduction
What is Special Ops? **10**
So You Want to be in Special Ops? **17**

Part II: The Special Ops 12-Week Workout
Stretches **37**
Upper Body Exercises **52**
Lower Body Exercises **66**
Abs/Core Exercises **80**
The Special Ops 12-Week Workout Schedule **89**

Part III: Advanced 6-Week Workouts
Workout Notes **108**
Army Ranger & Green Beret Workout **123**
Air Force PJ/CCT Workout **137**
Navy SEAL Workout **151**

Part IV: Special Ops Nutrition **165**

Appendix
Selected Special Ops Acronyms **191**
Recruiting Information **192**
About the authors **193**
GetFitNow.com Online Support **195**

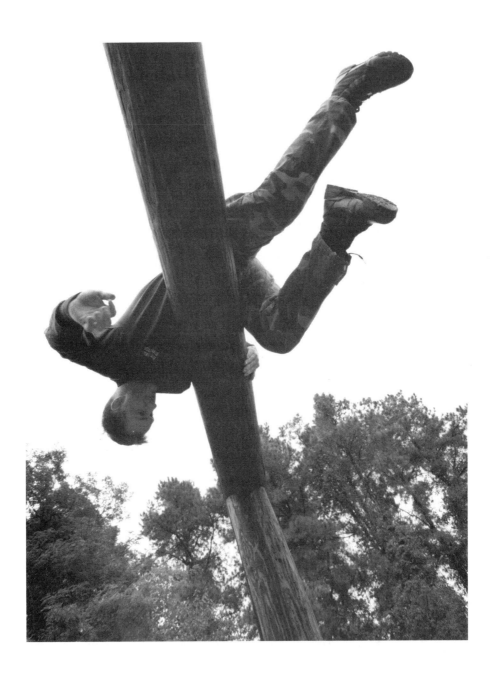

FOREWORD

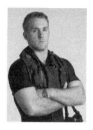

The Special Ops Workout encompasses all the types of workouts and exercises you will experience in any branch of Special Forces training. Whether you want to become a member of the Special Forces or you just want a challenging workout program, this book has something for you:

★ **A Baseline Fitness Program** for foundation building by Mike Mejia. This program will prepare you for Special Forces Physical Fitness Training (PT), including long runs, weight-bearing ruck marches, and miles of swimming with fins. It's also a great weight room workout for those who just want a change of pace.

★ **6-Week Army Ranger & Green Beret Workout** with PT, running, and load-bearing training

★ **6-Week Air Force PJ/CCT Workout** with special water skills training

★ **6-Week Navy SEAL Fitness Workout** with hard-core PT, running, and swimming

The Special Ops Workout isn't for everyone. Although the workout exercises require very little equipment, the number of reps, miles of running or swimming, and the sheer intensity of the workouts may be challenging for many. If you're a beginner or intermediate exerciser, I recommend you use the book as a guide and attempt only what you can do successfully. When you reach failure, stop. With these workouts, you will succeed by failing. Remember to keep trying! As you continue to perform these workouts, you will become stronger and able to reach the requirements of the Special Forces candidates.

Whether you want to enlist in the armed forces or just train to increase your strength and endurance, these workouts will get you in the best shape of your life. Good luck!

—Stew Smith, USN (SEAL)

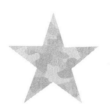

PART I:

INTRODUCTION

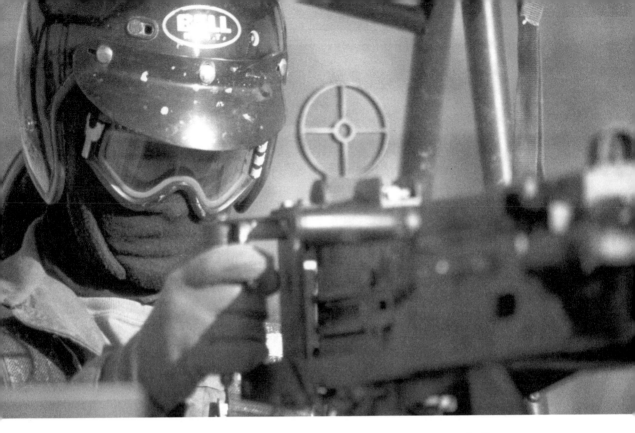

WHAT IS SPECIAL OPS?

SPECIAL OPERATIONS FORCES PERFORM POLITICALLY SENSITIVE missions that require the best equipped and most proficient forces. In these missions, it is of the utmost importance that deployed soldiers avoid detection and succeed in order to uphold U.S. prestige and interests.

The United States Special Operations Forces (SOF) is a joint task force of Army, Navy, and Air Force recruits that is commanded by the United States Special Operations Command (USSOCOM). Special Ops forces are uniquely trained and equipped with skills—called for in times of war and peace—not provided by other elements of the U.S. armed forces or the forces of other nations.

The elite SOF, which is comprised of a total active and reserve force of almost 46,000, can provide rapidly deployable and flexible joint task forces. In 1999, for example, SOF conducted engagement operations in over one hundred countries.

The USSOCOM prepares and maintains combat-ready SOF, which can quickly be deployed on challenging missions. These missions vary greatly in scope—from promoting peace and deterring aggression to providing humanitarian assistance and conducting combat operations.

The dedicated individuals of the SOF are mature and high-caliber professionals with intelligence, stamina, and well-developed problem-solving skills. Every day, these specially skilled, and highly trained, fit, and motivated soldiers must be ready to test their mental toughness as well as their physical endurance—they must be flexible, determined, and ready to face challenges with integrity and self-confidence.

HISTORY OF THE SPECIAL OPS

Special Operations have been a part of our military history since the colonial era. In fact, the United States has employed special operations tactics and strategies to exploit an enemy's vulnerabilities in every conflict since the Revolutionary War. These operations have always been carried out by specially trained people with a remarkable inventory of skills. In 1987, the creation of USSOCOM formally enhanced the ability of the United States to conduct special operations and engage in low-intensity conflict activities.

THE SPECIAL OPS TODAY

Today's SOF perform reconnaissance, psychological operations, and unconventional warfare in hot spots around the world. Using high-tech surveillance equipment, and modified aircraft and weapons, they participate in military operations such as Desert Shield and Desert Storm in the Middle East, Operation Urgent Fury in Grenada, and in humanitarian missions such as Operation Provide Promise, a relief effort in the Balkans.

Since September 11, 2001, Special Ops forces have played a key role in combating and deterring terrorism against the United States, deploying units in Afghanistan and Iraq.

In Iraq, Special Operations forces have played a key role in killing or capturing key Iraqi leaders, as well as taking command of Iraqi control facilities and means of

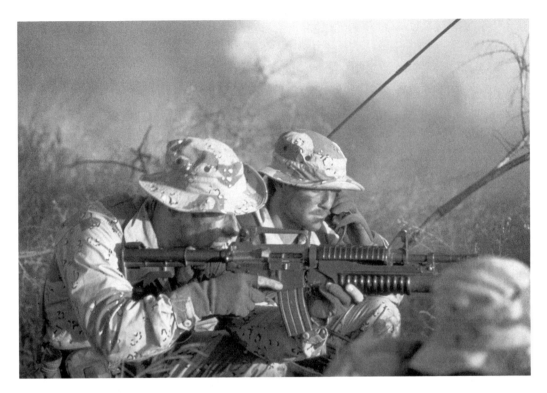

communications. Intelligence gathering will likely continue to be a critical function for the Special Ops units.

For the foreseeable future, the focus of Special Operations forces will continue to vary considerably by region. For example, in the Southern Command, consisting of Latin America, the Caribbean Sea, and the Gulf of Mexico, the focus is on drug production and trafficking, and enhancing regional stability. In Korea, the focus is on deterrence and readiness, particularly in the face of nuclear aggression.

SOF PRINCIPAL MISSIONS AND ACTIVITIES

SOF are usually broken down into small operational units made up of highly specialized men trained to use equipment designed specifically for each mission. The recruits in these special operational units train rigorously and their skills and capabilities greatly surpass those of conventional forces. Currently, the SOF are organized and trained in nine principal mission areas.

"Historians will likely view the Central Asian theater as Special Ops' finest hour. After the September 11 terrorists attacks, units deployed quickly to launching points in Uzbekistan and on the Navy carrier USS *Kitty Hawk*. Some units...stayed together for the battle. Other commandos were mixed-and-matched to fit the mission. An October raid on the home of Taliban leader Mullah Mohammed Omar featured Rangers, Green Berets, and elite Delta Force soldiers...in the bloody battles of Gardez, reconnaissance-in-force teams, on MH-47 Chinnook helicopters, brought in platoon-size units of Green Berets, Air Force air controllers and Navy SEALs."

June 2002: Soldier of Fortune, "U.S. Special Operations in Afghanistan", by Rowan Scarborough.

Because of the intense and specialized training SOF units undergo, they are frequently assigned to participate in non-SOF activities as well. These "collateral activities" vary depending on the changing international environment. Collateral activities of the SOF include Coalition support, combat research and rescue (CSAR), counter drug (CD) activities, and humanitarian assistance (HA), among others.

SOF IN TIMES OF PEACE

Special Operations Forces can help nations create the conditions necessary for stable development, which reduces the risk of armed conflict. By training a nation's own forces to provide their own security and educating them about Civil Affairs (CA) and Psychological Operations (PSYOP) programs, small SOF teams can help prevent local problems from developing into threats to internal and international stability. Soldiers work closely with the host nation government, military forces, and population to help them resolve their own problems. The work they do to resolve or contain regional conflicts or respond to natural disasters may in some cases prevent the need to deploy large conventional forces.

These same SOF teams often build strong relationships with the local military and civilian groups with whom they come in contact. These relationships can be of

SPECIAL OPERATIONS FORCES CAN:

★ Quickly organize and deploy tailored responses to many different situations

★ Gain entry to, and operate in, hostile or denied areas

★ Provide limited security and medical assistance for themselves and those they support

★ Communicate worldwide with unit equipment

★ Live in austere, harsh environments without extensive support

★ Survey and assess local situations and report quickly and efficiently

★ Work closely with host nation military and civilian authorities and populations

★ Organize indigenous people into working teams to help solve local problems

★ Deploy at relatively low cost, with a low profile and less intrusive presence than larger conventional forces

great importance to U.S. forces if they have to work later with these same organizations, either as coalition partners, or in localized combat operations.

Additionally, SOF contact with foreign military hierarchies provides an effective, low-cost way of cultivating respect for human rights and democratic values.

SOF IN TIMES OF WAR

In wartime, SOF conduct operational and strategic missions that support the joint force commander's (JFC's) campaign plan, either directly or indirectly. SOF missions originate with the JFC—often with the advice of the joint force special operations component commander (JFSOCC). Their goals are exactly the same as those of conventional forces. Special Operations Forces can help the JFC achieve decisive results by attacking operational and strategic targets and by carrying out PSYOP to deceive and demoralize the enemy. In addition, SOF work with local

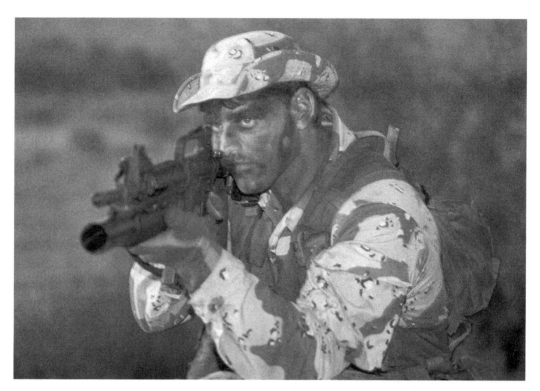

forces, helping them increase their contributions to the campaign plan. They also conduct coalition support to help integrate multinational forces into a cohesive, combined task force to carry out coalition goals. Additionally, CA and PSYOP can contribute directly to the commander's maneuverability by reducing the number of civilians on or near battlefield areas.

Additionally, Special Ops Forces play a vital role in post-conflict operations. Many of the same skills and talents used by SOF prior to and during combat situations are applicable after fighting has stopped. These forces can help establish (or re-establish) the infrastructure that is vital for a peaceful, prosperous society. Special Ops Forces training skills, coupled with CA and PSYOP expertise, help speed the return to normalcy, which allows conventional forces to quickly re-deploy. Special Ops Forces can also conduct stand-alone operations in situations where a small, discreet force provides the nation's leaders with options that fall somewhere between diplomatic efforts and the use of high-profile conventional forces.

Moreover, the relatively small size and capabilities of highly trained, joint SOF units enable them to react rapidly and provide the United States with options that limit the risk of escalation, which otherwise might accompany the commitment of larger conventional forces. Most often, these options include unconventional warfare, direct action, and special reconnaissance missions, such as insurgency, counterterrorism, counterdrug activities, surgical counterproliferation, and counterinsurgency.

Counterproliferation of weapons of mass destruction (WMD) is USSOCOM's highest operational priority. SOF can enhance the effectiveness of U.S. military, other government agencies, and international organizations in deterring proliferation of WMD and reacting appropriately if deterrence measures fail.

Against a growing security challenge, SOF offers a wide variety of skills to combat terrorism. One area of focus includes defensive antiterrorism measures, such as training and advising of security techniques, procedures, and systems that reduce vulnerability. The other major element of SOF operational capabilities centers on offensive counterterrorism measures directed at preventing, deterring, and vigorously responding to terrorist acts against U.S. interests, wherever they occur.

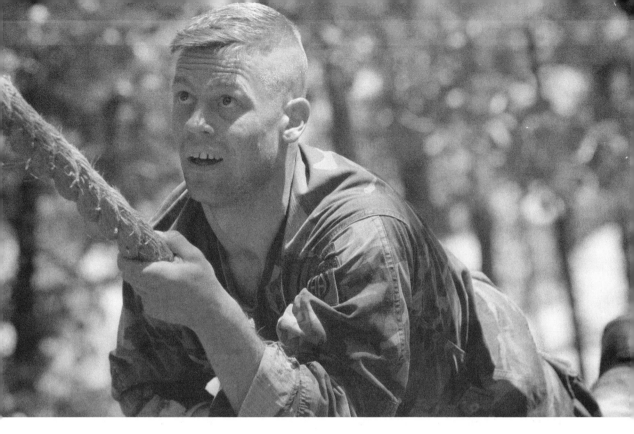

SO YOU WANT TO BE IN SPECIAL OPS?

THE CHARACTERISTICS OF SOF RECRUITS ARE SHAPED BY THE requirements of their missions. They may need to know foreign languages and understand different cultures or need training to use specialized equipment. SOF personnel must also have a firm grasp on the political context of each mission. All of these characteristics make SOF recruits unique in the U.S. military and enable them to work effectively with both civilians and other military forces.

Soldiers who want to join the SOF must undergo a rigorous testing and selection process. The reputation of the United States may rely on a mission being completed successfully, so only the most qualified, dependable, and self-reliant soldiers are chosen.

★ THE REAL DEAL: WHO'S GOING TO MAKE IT ★

"By far, the three physical abilities that are most key to success in Special Ops are running, swimming, and strength; particularly upper body strength.

You won't see very many body-building types in the Special Ops units, and my advice would be to avoid focusing on building muscle mass or looking good in the mirror. Most soldiers in Special Ops are lean, triathlon types, because of all the running and swimming they do."

—Dave Garcia
U.S. Army, 11th Group Special Forces

Each branch of the military has similar requirements—a basic physical test and oral examination—to apply to their Special Operations units.

ARMY

The Army component of the Special Ops is comprised of four major groups, all of which are governed by the U.S. Army Special Operations Command (USASOC). The USASOC makes sure that Special Ops forces are always ready and well equipped for all-weather and all-terrain environments. These soldiers are prepared for rapid deployment anywhere in the world.

The four major USASOC forces include:

Army Special Forces (Green Berets). In addition to the individual skills of operations and intelligence, communications, medical aid, engineering, and weapons, Army Special Forces soldiers can train, advise, and help host nation military or paramilitary forces. These soldiers are area-oriented; in other words, they are specially trained in their area's native language and culture. Green Berets have earned the nickname, "Quiet Professionals," and have been involved in peacetime operations and armed conflicts around the world over the past five decades.

Army Rangers. This strike force has taken part in every major U.S. combat operation since the end of the Vietnam War. Army Rangers fight primarily at night

ARMY PFT STANDARDS

Ranger and Green Beret students are challenged physically during training and should be able to perform above average in each of the following events before attending:

★ APFT (Army Physical Fitness Test)—Score 100 points in each event: Push-ups, sit-ups, and a 2-mile run
★ Pull-ups—Be able to do 10 to 20-plus deadhang
★ 5-Mile Run—Do in at least 35:00 to 40:00
★ 16-Mile Road March: 17:00 to 20:00 per mile
★ Land Navigation—Do ruck march / land navigation
★ Swim wearing your battle dress uniform (BDU) and gear.

and rely on elements of surprise, teamwork, and basic soldiering skills to undertake and accomplish special U.S. missions. Rangers can deploy rapidly by land, sea, or air.

Aviation—Night Stalkers. The 160th Special Operations Aviation Regiment is equipped with high-tech helicopters that have extremely accurate lift and attack capabilities and that can carry out a range of missions, including force insertion

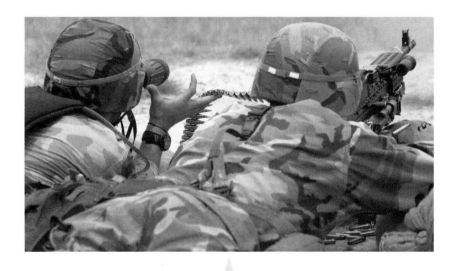

ARMY ELIGIBILITY REQUIREMENTS

Here are some of the basic qualifications you must meet to attend Army Special Ops training:

★ Be a male U.S. Citizen between 17 and 27 years of age
★ Be Airborne qualified
★ Meet specific physical fitness standards
★ Swim 50m in full BDU prior to Special Forces Assessment and Selection (SFAS)
★ Be a high school graduate or have a GED
★ Able to obtain a *secret* security clearance

and extraction, aerial security, and armed attack. These troops are world-renowned for the endurance and perseverance of its soldiers, who hold fast to their motto, "Night Stalkers Don't Quit."

Psychological Operations. These individuals receive extensive cross-cultural and language training that helps them once they are deployed. PSYOP units carry out operations that help "induce or reinforce attitudes and behaviors favorable to U.S. national goals" among foreign audiences. The PSYOP motto is "Persuade, Change, Influence." PSYOP forces often use print and broadcast media to carry out their missions.

ARMY SPECIAL FORCES TRAINING

The primary training ground for Special Forces is at the John F. Kennedy Special Warfare Center and School at Fort Bragg, North Carolina. Today's young recruits who want to wear the Green Beret begin their year-long training with the Special Forces Assessment and Selection (SFAS) course. This 4-week "prep" course is designed to screen, assess, and select soldiers for the Special Forces Qualification Course (SFQC) known as the "Q Course." (Many

Rangers attend this training, but it is not mandatory to be a Ranger before becoming a Green Beret).

The SFAS allows Special Forces instructors to assess each soldier by testing his physical, emotional, and mental stamina. The program assesses tactical skills, leadership, physical fitness, motivation, and ability to cope with stress (experienced by all soldiers) in a controlled and subjective environment. This phase helps reduce the drop-out rate by allowing only the most highly motivated soldiers to move on to the next phase of training, the Q Course. The SFAS also allows each soldier to make an educated decision about whether SF fits into his career plans.

After the SFAS, Green Beret training begins with **Phase One,** which lasts 40 days. In this phase, individual skills are assessed and taught. Such skills include map reading and land navigation, small units tactics and patrols, and survival in harsh environments. **Phase Two** of the Green Beret Q Course is specialty training, which lasts for 60 days.

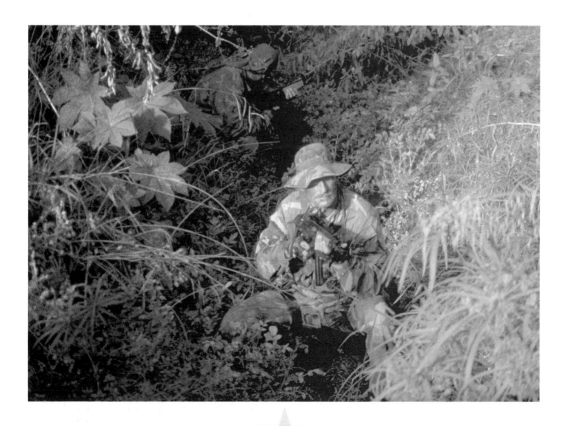

ARMY RANGER TRAINING

Army Rangers are taught at the renowned Ranger School in Fort Benning, Georgia. This extremely difficult 61-day training course for Special Operations soldiers is divided into three phases:

Benning Phase, designed to develop military skills, physical and mental endurance, and confidence. This phase also teaches the Ranger how to properly maintain himself and his equipment under difficult field conditions.

Mountain Phase, where the Ranger develops his ability to plan, prepare, and execute phases of all types of combat operations, including ambushes and raids, plus environmental and survival techniques.

Florida Phase, where further ability is developed in planning and leading small units on independent and coordinated airborne, air assault, amphibious, small boat and dismounted combat operations.

★ THE REAL DEAL: GETTING IN SHAPE ★

"If you feel that Special Ops is the career path for you, check it out; do as much research as you can, because there is a lot of useful information out there. Prepare yourself ahead of time.

If you are already in good shape, your journey will be much smoother. Most of the tests that measure your motivation are based around physical activity—under the assumption that if your mind gives out, you won't make it physically. Quitters compromise both the mission and their fellow soldiers."

—Dave Garcia
U.S. Army, 11th Group Special Forces

★ THE RANGER CREED ★

Command Sergeant Major Gentry wrote the Ranger Creed in 1974. Today, it is recited by Rangers during change of command ceremonies, regimental and battalion level physical training, upon graduation from Ranger school, and daily by young Rangers in the regiment.

"Recognizing that I volunteered as a Ranger, fully knowing the hazards of my chosen profession, I will always endeavor to uphold the prestige, honor and high 'esprit de corps' of my Ranger Regiment.

Acknowledging the fact that a Ranger is a more elite soldier who arrives at the cutting edge of battle by land, sea, or air. I accept the fact that as a Ranger my country expects me to move farther, faster, and fight harder than any other soldier.

Never shall I fail my comrades. I will always keep myself mentally alert, physically strong and morally straight and I will shoulder more than my share of the task whatever it may be. One hundred percent and then some.

Gallantly will I show the world that I am a specially selected and well-trained soldier. My courtesy to superior officers, neatness of dress and care of equipment shall set the example for others to follow.

Energetically will I meet the enemies of my country. I shall defeat them on the field of battle for I am better trained and will fight with all my might. Surrender is not a Ranger word. I will never leave a fallen comrade to fall into the hands of the enemy and under no circumstances will I ever embarrass my country.

Readily will I display the intestinal fortitude required to fight on to the Ranger objective and complete the mission, though I be the lone survivor."

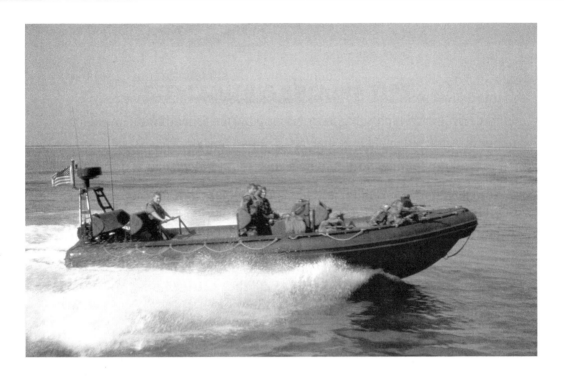

NAVY

The Navy contributes two elite groups—SEAL teams and Special Boat Squadrons—to Special Operations Forces. Both are commanded by the Naval Special Warfare Command (NAVSPECWARCOM), which is responsible for maintaining the readiness of active and reserve Naval Special Warfare (NSW) forces.

SEAL Teams. The history of Sea, Air, Land (SEAL) teams dates to the elite frogmen of World War II. These maritime multipurpose combat forces undergo extremely tough physical and mental training—in fact, SEALs are considered the best-trained combat swimmers in the world. SEALs are different from other Special Ops groups in that they are maritime special forces—they strike from and return to the sea. Their stealth and clandestine modes of operation mean they can conduct missions against targets that larger forces could not without being detected.

Special Boat (SB) Squadrons are composed of specially trained naval personnel who can operate and maintain a variety of special operations ships and

NAVY SEAL PFT STANDARDS

★ 500-yard swim using the side or breaststroke (12:30 minimum, 7:00 to 8:30 competitive range)
★ 10-minute rest
★ Maximum number of push-ups in 2:00 (42 minimum, 100 to 120 competitive range)
★ 2-minute rest
★ Maximum number of sit-ups in 2:00 (50 minimum, 100 to 120 competitive range)
★ 2-minute rest
★ Maximum number of pull-ups (8 minimum, 20 to 30 competitive range)
★ 10-minute rest
★ 1.5-mile run in boots and pants (11:30 minimum, 8:30 to 10:00 competitive range)

NAVY SEAL ELIGIBILITY REQUIREMENTS

★ Be a male, U.S. citizen
★ Be 28 years old or younger. Waivers for men ages 29 to 30 are granted on a case-by-case basis.
★ Have vision of no worse than 20/40 in one eye and 20/70 in the other, and it must be correctable to 20/20 with no color blindness. You may have a waiver if vision is 20/70 in one eye and 20/100 in the other, correctable to 20/20. A waiver is also necessary for people who have Photorefractive Keratectomy (PRK) surgery before enlisting.
★ Meet specific physical fitness standards
★ Be a high school graduate or have a GED

crafts. SB units can provide strategic mobility by conducting coastal and river-based missions.

NAVY SEAL TRAINING

Navy-based Special Ops Forces are trained at the Naval Special Warfare Center at Coronado, California. There, SEAL recruits undergo Basic Underwater Demolition/SEAL (BUD/S) training . The intense training is split into three phases:

Basic conditioning, an eight-week course of physical conditioning, including running, swimming and calisthenics. Trainees also learn small boat seamanship in this phase.

Diving, a seven-week phase that concentrates on scuba training.

Land warfare, a physically intense 10-week training phase with a focus on demolition, reconnaissance, weapons, and tactics. Students learn land navigation, small-unit tactics, rappelling, military land, and underwater explosives, and weapons training.

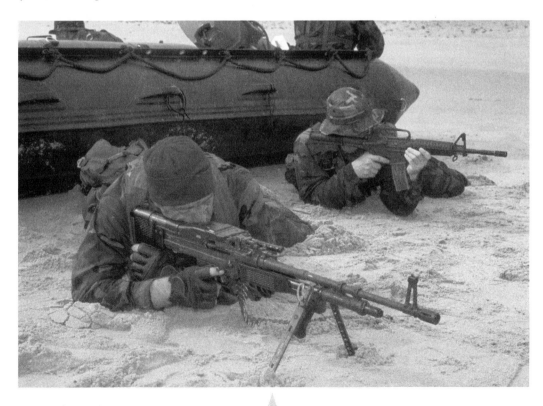

★ **THE REAL DEAL: FEAR** ★

"The most difficult challenge for many soldiers is overcoming basic fears—you're jumping out of planes, diving into cold water, testing yourself physically in ways you've never done before, over and over again. If anyone ever says that they are not afraid in a situation like that, they are either lying or crazy. Fear can be positive for a soldier, because it keeps you from hurting yourself—but too much fear provokes a sensory overload. You need to keep a good balance. There are many unknown variables in every situation, but you can't dwell on them. At the same time your sense of fear helps you maintain your senses so you can react if something does go wrong."

—**Dave Garcia**
U.S. Army, 11th Group Special Forces

AIR FORCE

The Air Force Special Operations Command (AFSOC) makes sure active Air Force Reserve and Air National Guard SOF are prepared for rapid deployment anywhere in the world. Air Force SOF are specialists in unconventional warfare, psychological operations, special reconnaissance, civil affairs, combating terrorism, and foreign internal defense. Three special operations wings, two special operations groups, and one special tactics group are assigned to AFSOC.

Pararescue (PJs). The primary mission of pararescue, or parajumpers, is personnel recovery and emergency medical capabilities in peacetime and combat environments. The official motto of the Air Force Pararescue unit is, "These things we do, that others may live."

Combat Control Technicians (CCTs). CCTs, whose motto is "First there", play a vital role in combat situations. CCTs, trained to insert into any terrain and environment, provide ground force commanders with vital communications and essential command and control links for combat aircraft.

AIR FORCE TRAINING

Air Force soldiers of the SOF receive intensive training at the Air Force Special Operations School at Hurlburt Field, Florida. Training covers a wide range of deployment capabilities, including:

★ Parachute operations in low/high altitudes (into forests, water)

★ Waterborne infiltrations (scuba, aircraft boat drops, surface swimming)

★ Mountain operations (rock and ice climbing, rappelling, high angle evacuations)

★ Helicopter operations (rappelling, fast rope, rope ladder, hoist operations, gunner/scanner)

★ Overland movement (motorcycles, all-terrain vehicles, motor vehicles, team navigation)

★ Arctic operations (cross-country skiing, downhill skiing, snow mobilers, snowshoes, arctic sleds)

The school also gives instruction in in aviation foreign internal defense (FID), crisis response management, joint PSYOP, and revolutionary warfare.

AIR FORCE PJ/CCT PFT STANDARDS

The Physical Ability and Stamina Test (PAST) consists of the following:

★ Run 1.5 miles in 10:30 minutes or less

★ Swim 1000 meters, side or freestyle stroke, in 26:00 minutes or less

★ Swim 25 meters underwater without resurfacing

★ Complete 8 chin-ups in 1:00 minute or less

★ Complete 50 sit-ups in 2:00 minutes or less

★ Complete 50 push-ups in 2:00 minutes or less

★ Complete 50 flutter kicks in 2:00 minutes or less

AIR FORCE PJ/CCT ELIGIBILITY REQUIREMENTS

To be eligible to become a PJ or CCT, you must:

★ Be a U.S. citizen between 17 and 27 years old
★ Be a volunteer
★ Be a male
★ Be able to pass a Class III flight physical (done during basic training)
★ Have vision of no worse than 20/100, correctable to 20/20
★ Have normal color vision
★ Be able to obtain a secret security clearance (done during basic training)
★ Meet specific physical fitness standards
★ Be a high school graduate or have a GED
★ Attain a score of at least 100 points on the PAST, to be completed during basic training
★ Be a proficient swimmer

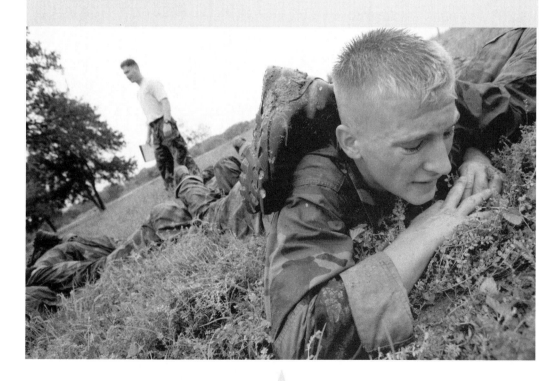

SPECIAL OPS TRAINING

After they are selected for training, candidates undergo extensive training in individual combat skills, foreign languages, and technical specialties required. They next move to a SOF aircrew, team, or squad for unit training. This is followed by cross-training in essential, special skills and advanced techniques.

Teamwork is emphasized throughout SOF training. In a team, all members must work well together; each must know the strengths, capabilities, and weaknesses of all of the other team members; and all must share a common doctrine that allows precise communication with minimal ambiguity.

Throughout this process, physical fitness training is critical. SOF need to be extremely fit and agile and have maximum endurance because their missions often take place in harsh climates, over extended periods of time, without conventional support and require frequent, quick adjustments to new environments. In addition, SOF training also includes regional orientation, which ensures that soldiers understand the culture, political climate, and language of the regions in which they will operate.

SOF training takes place in all kinds of terrain, in all climates, and continuously. Units may move from cold weather training in Alaska to ski training in New Hampshire to desert training in the Southwest. SOF are trained in urban combat, too, participating in shooting simulations at training facilities designed specifically for that purpose.

Even when they're not training in a specific environment, soldiers are still extremely physically active—running and swimming for several hours three to five times per week. And units that require para-jumping or scuba diving certification are tested frequently to remain certified.

Throughout training, SOF combine basic military and specialized skills training along with education. The goal of training is produce individuals units that have mastered the tactics, techniques, and procedures required to successfully perform their missions. In SOF training, soldiers learn the art and science of war and peacetime operations, and develop military judgment they need to creatively solve problems and deal with challenges. SOF training encourages innovation and demands that individuals think independently and use their own judgment.

★ THE REAL DEAL: MINDSET ★

In my opinion, the three most necessary mental characteristics are:
Discipline. No matter what kind of exhaustion or discomfort you experience, you keep going.
Focus. The ability to set your sights on a goal and attain it.
Commitment. To doing the best you can and fulfilling your goal.

If you are highly motivated, with the characteristics above, we can teach you the rest. You can work on your shooting skills or swimming skills or endurance levels. It's much, much harder to teach discipline and commitment. Half the battle is wanting to be there. The rest is having the knowledge to get you through any situation.

Special Ops soldiers have to be physically tough, which usually means that they are mentally tough as well. You need to have confidence in yourself and your abilities, combined with the desire to test yourself. You may not have that confidence when you enter the unit, but you won't know what you can truly accomplish until you try. The word "quit" was never in my vocabulary; I would think about ways to adapt instead.
—Dave Garcia
U.S. Army, 11th Group Special Forces

★ STEW SMITH ON MENTAL TOUGHNESS ★

Mental toughness! How do you get it? Are you born with it? Can you acquire it? Arguments about this question have occurred long before there was Special Operations training. I believe that mental toughness is borne of physical training, proper mindset, and a high level of maturity. This toughness is what propels you through long days of ruck marches without food, times when hours of being awake turn into days, when the pain of a nagging injury can be ignored. How do you get that?

Consider five-time Tour de France winner, Lance Armstrong, who beat cancer. After his battle with the deadly disease, he came back mentally tougher and has been at the top of his game ever since. Maybe he had it all along, who knows?

Mental toughness is not measurable; it is completely internal. But I believe that hard work will get you there. When Lance Armstrong was asked recently by reporters "What are you on?" referring to performance enhancing drugs. Lance stated, "I am on my bike!—busting my ass for six hours a day!"

The question is, do you get mental toughness by attending Special Ops training schools or by the training you do beforehand? The answer is a combination of both. I feel I was mentally tough because of the way I trained before attending SEAL training; I further developed my mental toughness to emerge feeling I was truly capable of anything and would not quit—ever.

I have seen *many* great athletes not graduate BUD/S and a *few* men who were not in very great shape graduate through sheer determination and daily gut checks. The few who graduated had a common trait, the ability to "play with pain," and a mental determination never to quit on themselves or—most importantly—their BUD/S classmates. Playing team sports in high school probably helped. Men who participated in sports in which playing with pain was required, such as wrestling, football, lacrosse, and others, usually did quite well.

The key? Arrive ready to compete, not merely to survive. This is the biggest difference between those who graduate any special forces training and those who do not. You should be in the type of shape that will allow you to win or be in the top 10 percent of the class in every event. If you can easily surpass the minimum standards (if not double them in pull-ups, push-ups, and sit-ups) on the respective PFTs, you will be in the top 10 percent of your class. You may be surprised by how many of your peers will barely pass the PFT on day one. This is true of the majority of graduates when they arrive at any SF school.

All this doesn't mean you will graduate if you can ace the standards. In fact, many Special Ops students with maximum scores have quit. Once you physically ace the PFT, it's mental toughness that will help you graduate. That is an immeasurable element of the Special Ops student. However, a common denominator among most of the graduates who have mental toughness is that they were also in great shape and did not mind being yelled at by instructors. Finding humor in what happens to you daily is one of the best ways to get through the grind.

Everyone at Special Ops training has a nemesis or weakness. For instance, great swimmers and guys with great upper body strength are usually poor runners. Big guys over 200 pounds also tend to have a difficult time running and getting through the obstacle course. Little guys who have wrestled usually don't have a problem with the running and obstacle course; but they're typically not great swimmers and can't carry heavy ruck sacks easily. Every now and then you will find someone who is great at all the events, but usually even he has a weakness and must push himself harder to win.

In your journey to find mental toughness, remember to train smart and not push yourself to injury that will require medical attention. Rehab is a long and slow process that will delay your efforts significantly.

—Stew Smith, USN (SEAL)

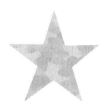

PART II:

SPECIAL OPS 12-WEEK WORKOUT

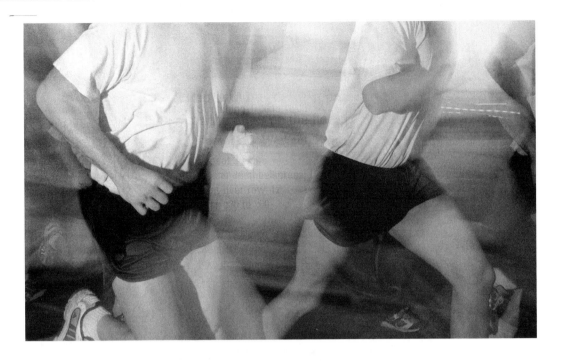

SPECIAL OPS 12-WEEK PROGRAM DESIGN

The following workout program follows a 12-week schedule, divided into three 4-week sections, combining weight training and conditioning. Phase I of the workout focuses on developing a strong conditioning foundation that will prepare you for the weeks to come. Phase II, weeks 5 through 8, will help stimulate muscle growth. In the final phase, weeks 9 through 12, the focus will be on refining your overall physical conditioning, to achieve true physical excellence in the spirit of the Special Ops Forces.

A 15-minute warm-up walk or jog is recommended before and after each workout to ensure that your muscles are loose and your mind is focused on the work ahead. Follow your warm-up jog with stretching exercises (5 to 10 minutes) that will help prevent injury and maximize the impact of the workout.

A final word: always consult your doctor or a medical professional when beginning a new workout. Remember, while it's great to feel the burn from lifting or conditioning, no exercise program should cause pain. Pain during the workout is a clear signal from your body to postpone your workout until your body can recover.

★ ★ ★ ★ ★ ★ ★ ★ ★ ★ ★ ★ ★ ★

STRETCHES

For a Special Operations Forces soldier, even a small injury can jeopardize the success of the mission—or even be life-threatening. All soldiers know that even though stretching can be tedious (especially when you're pumped to get to the "real" workout), it is by far the most effective way to prevent injury and prepare your body for the grueling workout to come.

Stretch for at least 15 minutes before and after your workout. It's not a bad idea to preface your stretching routine with a quick jog for one to two miles, or even 10 minutes of jumping jacks if you're pressed for time. This will help loosen your joints, raise your heart rate, and focus your mind.

Also keep in mind that proper technique during stretching is important to make sure your stretches are effective. Even if you're a seasoned athlete, this chapter is a good refresher on the types of stretches that will prepare you for a Special Ops workout.

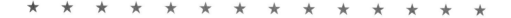

★ ★ ★ ★ ★ ★ ★ ★ ★ ★ ★ ★ ★ ★

NECK ROTATIONS

Start Position: Standing

Rotate your neck to the right, left, back and center, slowly and gently. Hold each position for 3-5 seconds before moving to the next position.

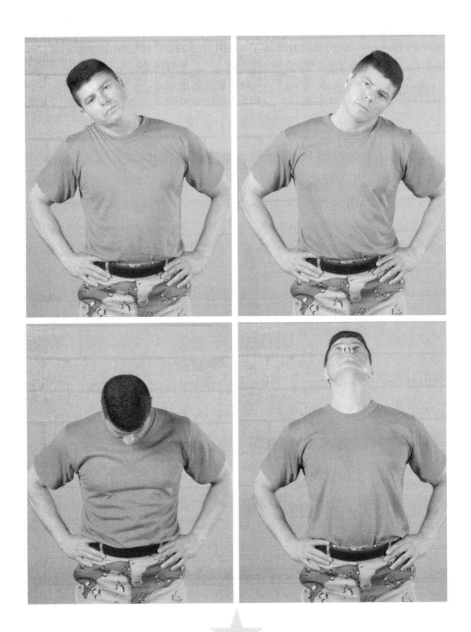

ARM CIRCLES

Start Position: Standing

Rotate your arms slowly in a large circle as shown, first going clockwise for 15 seconds, then counter-clockwise for the same duration.

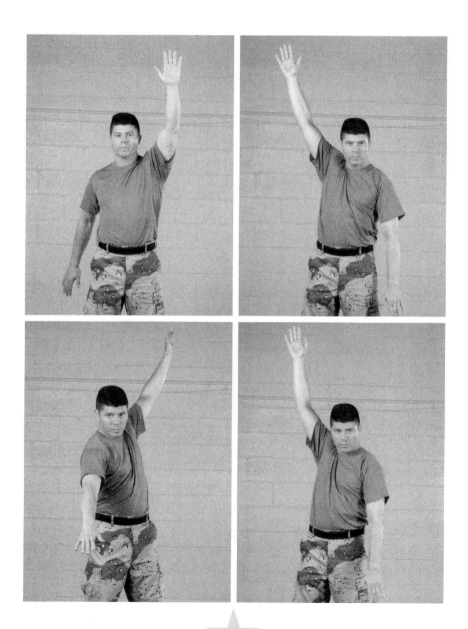

ARM / SHOULDER STRETCH

Start Position: Standing

Drop your shoulder and pull your arm across your chest as shown. Using the opposite arm, gently pull your straightened arm across your chest and hold for 15 seconds. Repeat with the other arm.

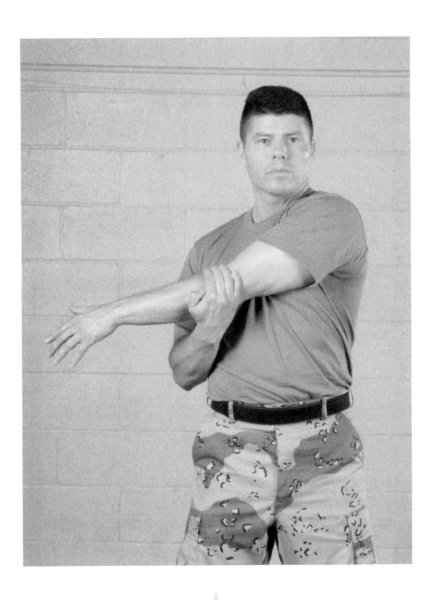

TRICEPS INTO BACK STRETCH

Start Position: Standing

Place both arms over and behind your head as shown. Grab your right elbow with your left hand and pull your elbow toward your opposite shoulder, leaning your body with the pull. Repeat with the other arm.

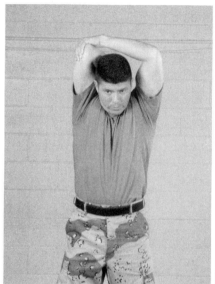
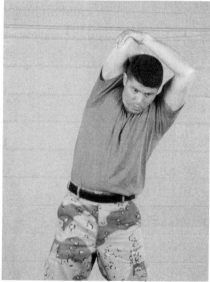

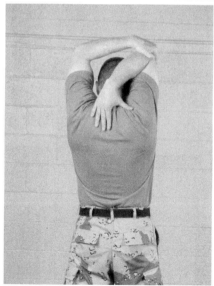

SWIMMER STRETCH

Start Position: Standing

Stand with your arms extended and parallel to the floor. Slowly pull your elbows back as far as you can and interlock your fingers. Pull your shoulders back and extend your chest. Hold for 15 seconds. Now reverse the stretch, bowing your back and rolling your shoulders forward, caving in your chest. This stretches the opposing muscle groups of the chest and upper back.

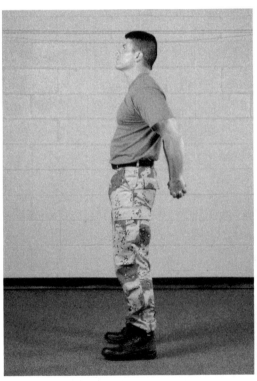 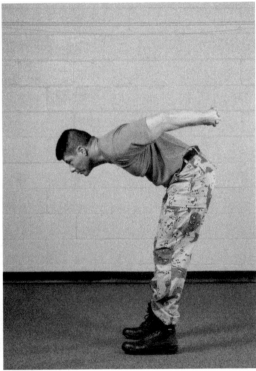

HAMSTRING STRETCH

Start Position: Standing or sitting

From the standing or sitting position, bend forward at the waist and touch your toes. Keep your back straight and slightly bend your knees. You should feel the muscles in the back of your thighs stretching.

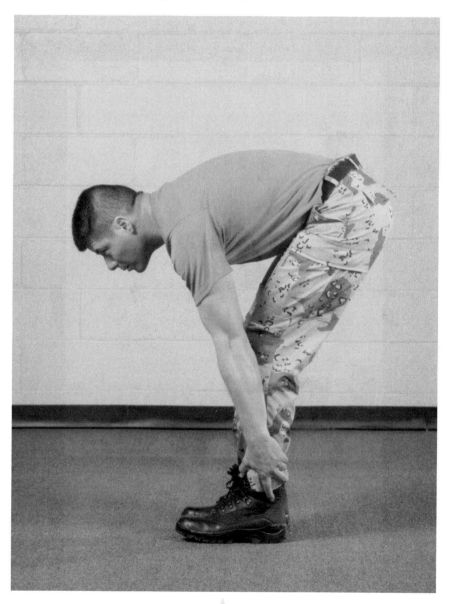

INNER THIGH SIDE STRETCH

Start Position: Standing

Stand with your legs spread and lean to the right, as shown. Keep the foot of the straightened leg pointing forward and the bent leg pointed in the direction the knee is bending. Repeat with the opposite leg.

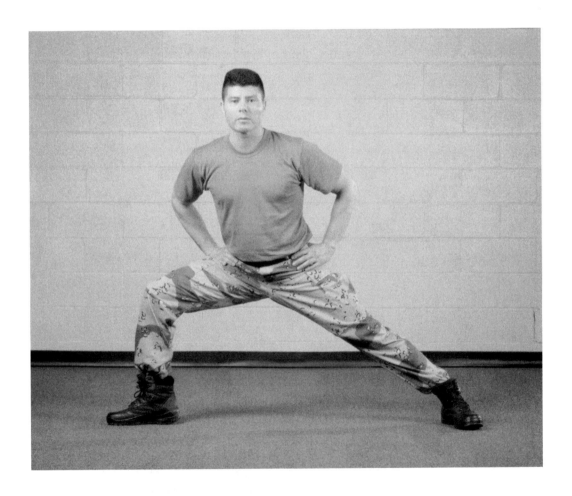

THIGH STRETCH STANDING

Start Position: Standing

Bend your knee and grab your foot at the ankle. Pull your heel to your buttocks and push your hips forward. Keep your knees close together and focus on tightening the muscles in the buttocks. Hold for 10-15 seconds and repeat with the other leg. (If needed, hold a chair or wall for balance, or lie down on your side to perform this stretch.)

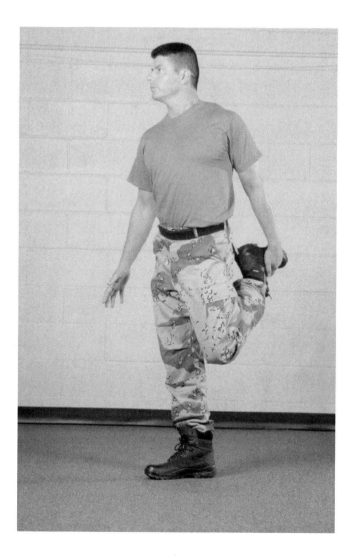

CALF STRETCH INTO ACHILLES TENDON STRETCH

Start Position: Standing

Stand with one foot 2 to 3 feet in front of the other. With both feet pointing in the direction you are facing, put most of your body weight on the back leg, stretching the calf muscle.

Now, bend the rear knee slightly, and you should feel the stretch in your heel.

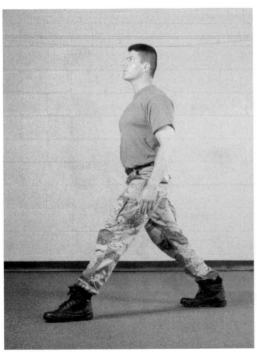 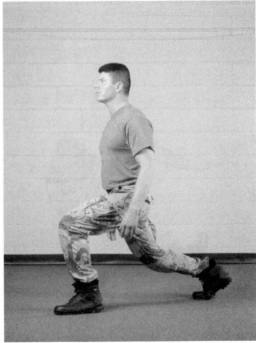

ABDOMINAL STRETCH

Start Position: Lying, on the stomach

From the start position, push yourself up to your elbows. Slowly lift your head and shoulders and look up at the sky or ceiling. Hold for 15 seconds and repeat twice.

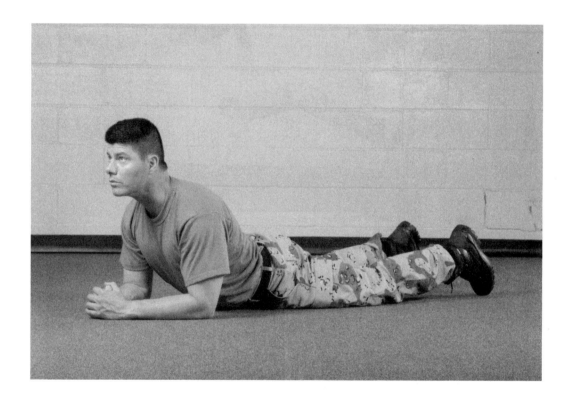

LOWER BACK STRETCH I

Start Position: Sitting

Sit on your knees in a fetal position as shown. Try to bring your head as close to your knees as possible. Put your chin to your chest and hold for 10 seconds. This helps stretch the muscles in the upper back and base of the neck.

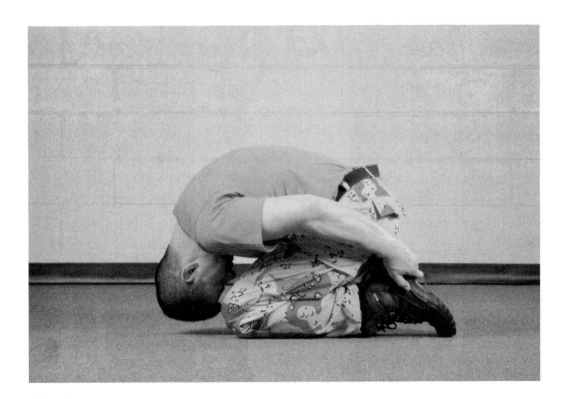

LOWER BACK STRETCH II

Start Position: Lying, on your side

From the start position on the right side, extend your top leg in front of you. Slowly twist your torso until your shoulders touch the floor. Hold for 15 seconds and repeat on the left side.

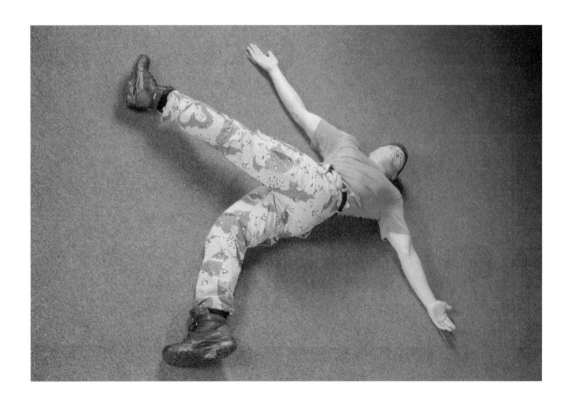

ILIOTIBIAL BAND (ITB) STRETCH I

Start Position: Sitting, with legs crossed in front of you

From the start position, and keeping your legs crossed, bring the top leg to your chest and bend it at the knee so that your foot is placed outside of your opposite leg's thigh. Hold your knee for 15 seconds against your chest and repeat with the other leg.

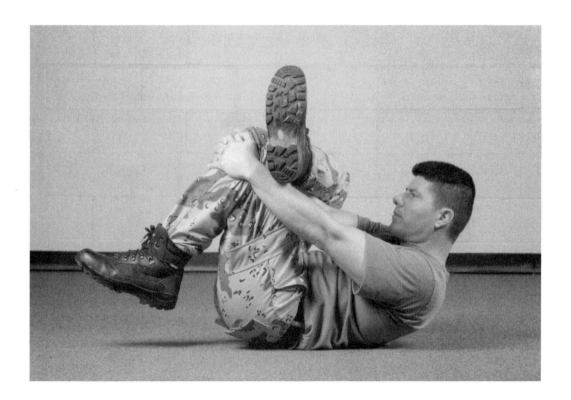

ITB STRETCH II

Start Position: Sitting

Sit with your left leg crossed over your right leg. Grab the right leg with both hands around the thigh or shin (with leg bent) and pull toward your chest. Repeat with the other leg.

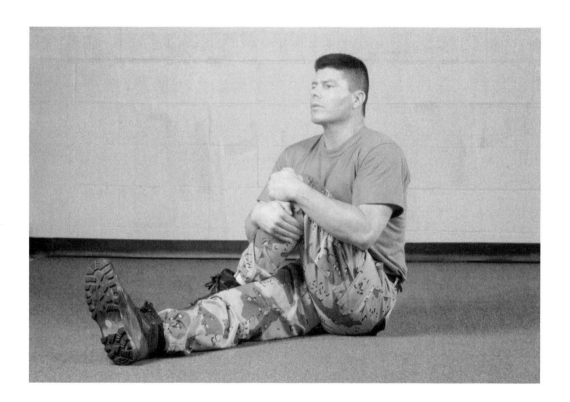

★ ★ ★ ★ ★ ★ ★ ★ ★ ★ ★ ★ ★ ★

UPPER BODY EXERCISES

★ ★ ★ ★ ★ ★ ★ ★ ★ ★ ★ ★ ★ ★

3-POINT PUSH-UP

Start Position: Standard push-up position

From the standard push-up position, "stack" one foot on top of the other to increase the difficulty level.

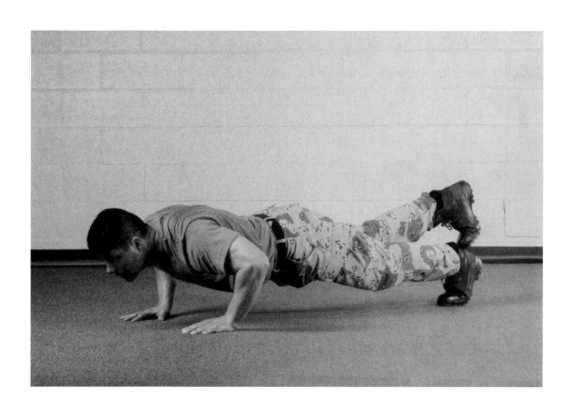

DIPS

Start Position: At dip bar, raised with arms locked

From the locked position, begin to lower yourself downward, leaning forward. Lower yourself until the backs of your arms are parallel or slightly beyond parallel to the floor. When you reach the bottom position, immediately begin to press your body upward without using any momentum. During the exercise, focus on working the chest and triceps muscles.

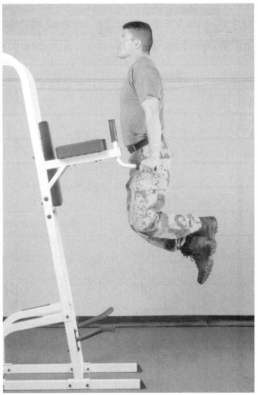
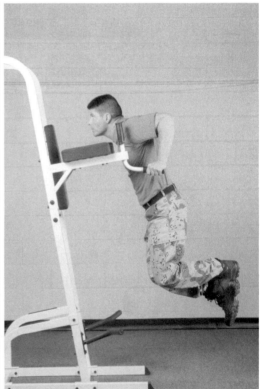

INCLINE DUMBBELL PRESS

Start Position: Lying on a bench, with dumbbells
Position the dumbbells out to the side of your chest, keeping your elbows wide and your forearms perpendicular to the floor. With the chest in its elevated position, press the dumbbells up toward the ceiling. As you reach the top of the exercise, you can either touch the dumbbells together or press them straight up like a bench press.

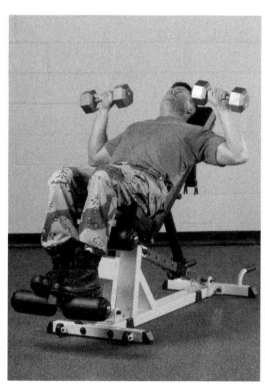 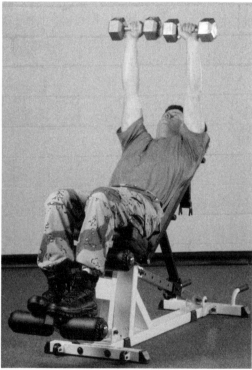

CHEST PRESS

Position: Lying on an exercise bench, with dumbbells

Place your feet shoulder-width apart and keep your back on the bend. Hold a dumbbell in each hand with your elbows bent at a 90-degree angle. Extend your arms toward the ceiling, but don't let the weights touch. Return to the starting position and repeat.

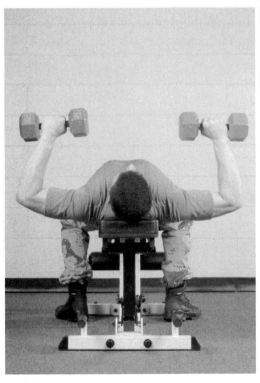 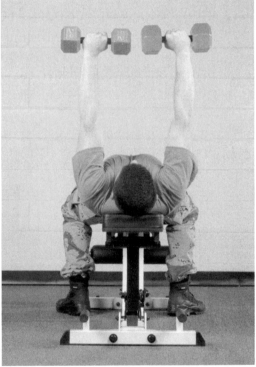

PIKE PUSH-UP

Start Position: Standard push-up position

Modify the standard push-up position so that your buttocks are up high in the air, and your body forms an inverted "V." Keeping your legs straight, bend your elbows and lower your head and shoulders toward the floor. When your face is just an inch or two from the floor, pause momentarily and push back up.

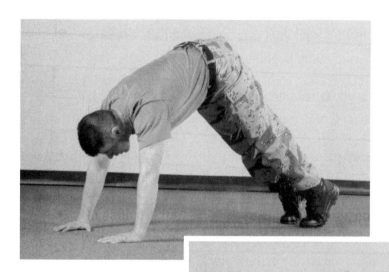

PLYO PUSH-UP

Start Position: Standard push-up position

Assume a push-up position and then rapidly lower yourself toward the floor. Before you actually touch the floor, immediately thrust yourself back up until your hands come a couple of inches off the ground. "Catch" yourself and immediately lower back down and repeat.

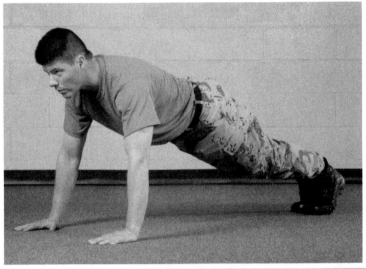

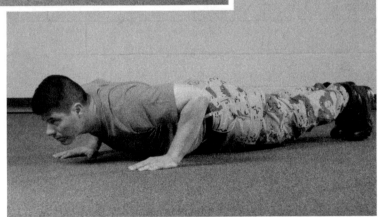

BENT-OVER ROW

Start Position: Standing, with dumbbells

Align your feet about shoulder width apart, making sure your knees are pointing directly in front of you throughout the movement. Bend over at the hips, making sure that your lower back is not slumped over. Stick out your chest while slightly squeezing your shoulder blades together. Begin rowing the elbows up toward the ceiling, allowing the back of the arms to lead the motion.

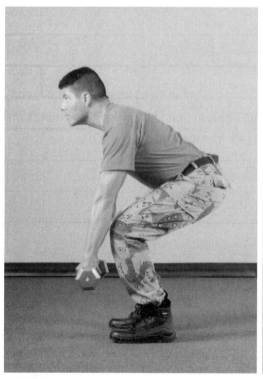 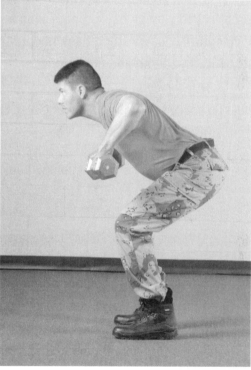

ROMANIAN DEADLIFT AND BENT-OVER ROW

Start Position: Standing, with dumbbells

Begin by executing a standard Romanian Deadlift, as follows: Stand with your feet shoulder width apart and knees slightly bent. Keeping your torso straight and tall, lift one foot an inch or two off the floor. Once you feel balanced, maintain a slight bend in the other knee as you slowly lean forward by sticking your hips back and bringing your torso over toward the floor. As you descend, be sure to maintain the arch in your lower back. Once your torso is almost parallel to the floor, pause momentarily before lifting back up into the start position.

Now, to add an additional twist:

Once in the bottom position, keep your elbows out to the sides as you row the dumbbells up until they touch your lower chest. Pause for a second before lowering them until your arms are straight and then press your heels into the floor to stand back up.

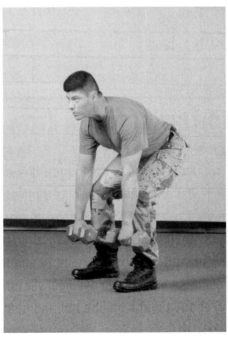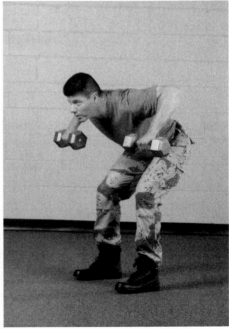

TOWEL PULL-UPS

Start Position: At the pull-up bar, with towel

Loop a towel over a standard pull-up bar. Grasp the ends of the towel in your hands, hang, and then execute a pull-up until your chin is over the bar. Pause, lower, and repeat.

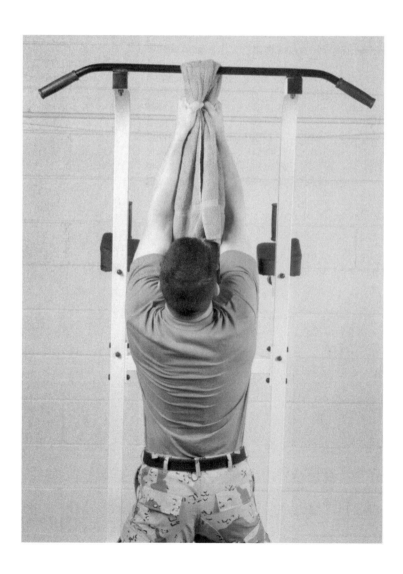

STAGGERED PULL-UPS

Start Position: Standing, at pull-up bar

This exercise is a pull-up with one arm set at a shoulder's width grip and the other about twice that wide, to provide an extra challenge for your upper body.

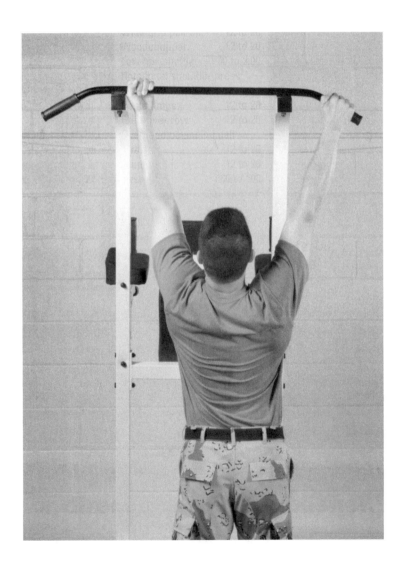

SUPERMANS

Start Position: Lying on the floor, face down

From the start position, extend your arms straight out in front of you and your legs straight out behind you. Keeping your arms and legs perfectly straight, simultaneously lift your arms, chest, and legs a few inches off the mat. Once there, hold the position for a second or two before lowering again. Repeat for the desired number of reps.

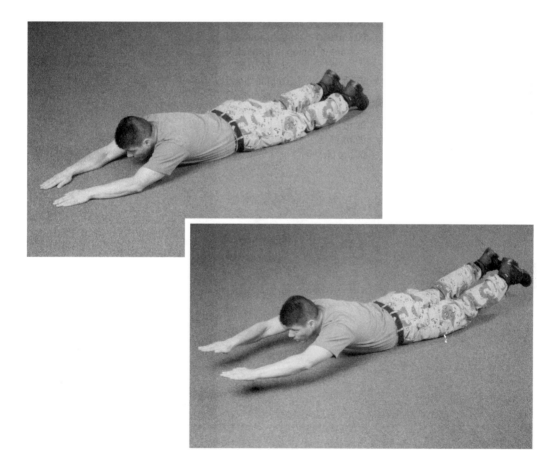

HANG CLEANS

Start Position: Standing, with dumbbells

Stand holding dumbbells at arm's length in front of you. Bend your knees and lean forward slightly so that the dumbbells are aligned with your lower thighs. Driving through your hips, knees, and ankles, rapidly accelerate the dumbbells upward as you simultaneously shrug, lift onto your toes, and upright row them toward the ceiling. Once the dumbbells are at about chest level, quickly flip them and drop under them as you catch them across your shoulders with your arms parallel to the floor. Return to the starting position and repeat.

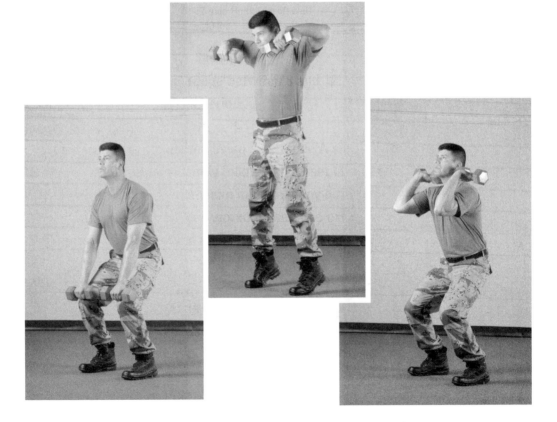

ROTATIONAL SHOULDER PRESS

Start Position: Standing, with dumbbells

This exercise is similar to the standard dumbbell shoulder press except that you rotate your torso as you press the dumbbells up, ending up turned completely to one side. Return to the start position and repeat.

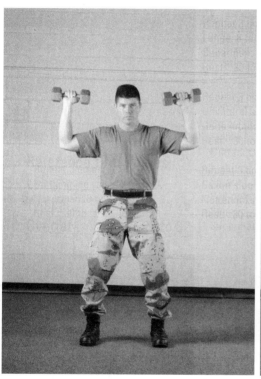 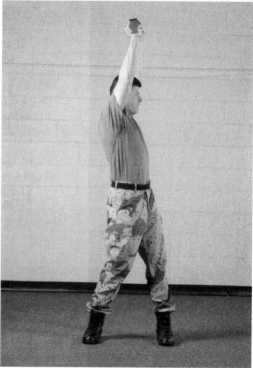

★ ★ ★ ★ ★ ★ ★ ★ ★ ★ ★ ★ ★ ★

LOWER BODY EXERCISES

★ ★ ★ ★ ★ ★ ★ ★ ★ ★ ★ ★ ★ ★

THE "BEAR"

Start Position: Standing, with dumbbells

Begin by lifting the dumbbells up to your shoulders. Once in the "rack" position, keep your upper arms parallel to the floor as you execute a front squat until the tops of your thighs are parallel to the floor. After returning to the standing position, quickly dip down and bend your knees slightly to generate the necessary momentum to explosively press the dumbbells over your head. Finish by lowering the dumbbells back to the shoulders and then back down across your thighs.

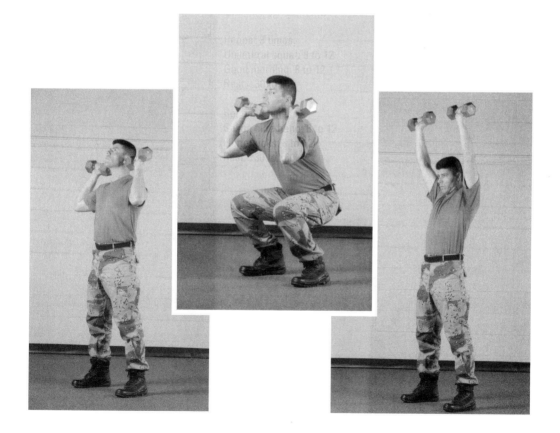

LOW BOX SHUFFLE

Start Position: Standing, with box or crate

For this one you'll need a step or sturdy crate approximately 12 inches high. Begin with one foot on the step and the other on the floor as you stand to one side of the step. Quickly step up sideways onto the box with one leg and down with the other. Repeat for 90 to 120 seconds.

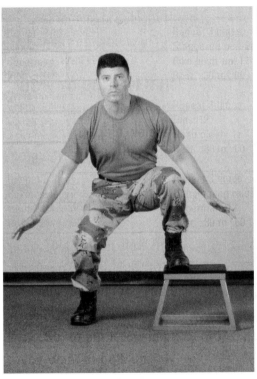
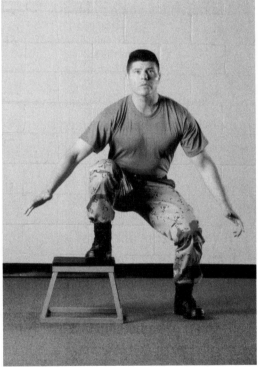

DUMBBELL SQUAT

Start Position: Standing, with dumbbells

Stand with feet shoulder width apart and knees slightly bent, holding a pair of dumbbells at your sides. Keeping your chest up and a slight arch in your lower back, squat down until the tops of your thighs are parallel to the floor. Pause for a second and press back up.

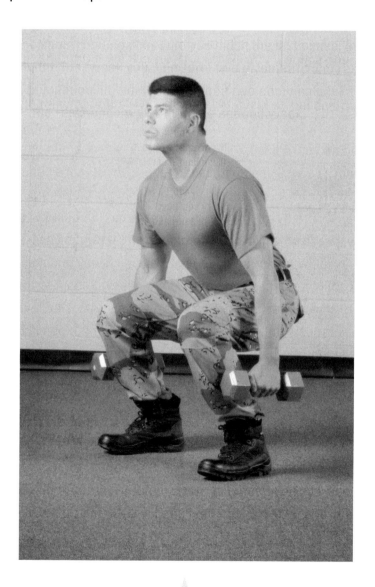

LUNGES

Start Position: Standing, with dumbbells

From the start position, step forward with your right foot. Bend at the knee making sure you descend slowly and in control. As your knee bends and your hips are lowering, lower yourself until your left knee is about two inches from the ground and stop. Begin to reverse the movement by pressing off the right foot only, to maximize the impact on the muscles. Return to the start position and immediately lunge with the left foot.

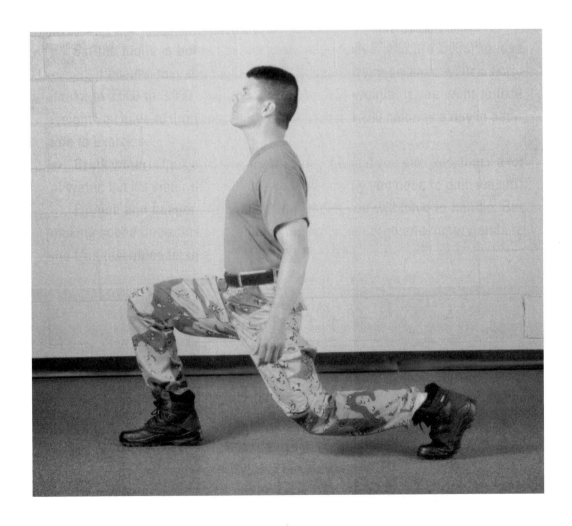

LUNGE JUMPS

Start Position: Standing

Assume a lunge position with your feet spread about 2 to 3 feet apart from front to back. Rapidly dip down by bending your knees and swinging your arms back behind you. Reverse directions quickly and swing your arms forward as you spring into the air. Once in the air, switch your front and back legs before landing for the next jump and continuing.

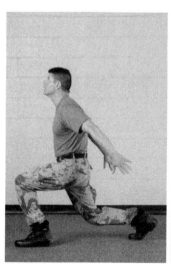
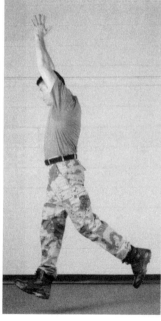
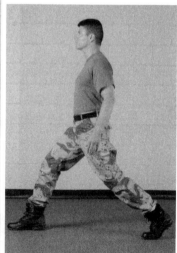

PENTA LUNGE

Start Position: Standing, with dumbbells

Hold a pair of dumbbells at your sides and begin by executing a standard forward lunge. After pushing back up to the starting position immediately lunge out at a 45-degree angle going forward. This motion is followed by a side lunge, a reverse lunge at a 45-degree angle, and a regular reverse lunge. A complete cycle as described above counts as one rep.

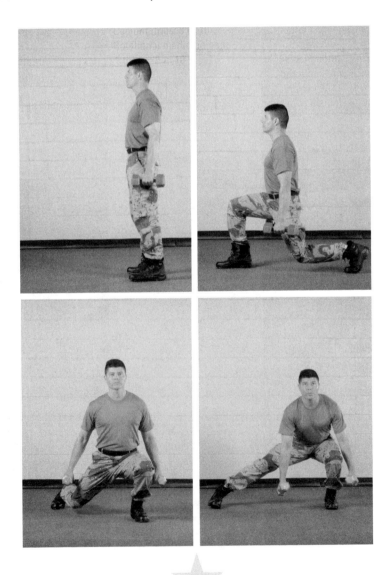

TRAVELING LUNGES

Start Position: Standing

Traveling lunges use the same principles as dumbbell lunges, but rely on continuous motion to increase the impact of the exercise on the leg muscles. Start on one side of the room and lunge forward with your right foot. However, instead of returning to the start position, continue lunging, moving forward with your left foot, until you reach the other side of the room or desired distance.

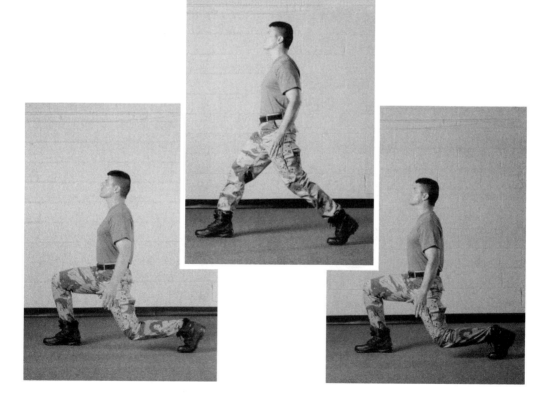

OVERHEAD BALANCING CALF RAISE

Start Position: Standing, with dumbbells

This exercise is similar to a standard calf raise, with the added challenge of holding dumbbells directly overhead. Use a wide or "snatch" grip. A snatch grip is a grip that wraps your index finger over your thumb to increase core stability and improve balance.

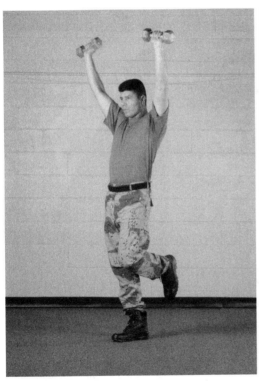 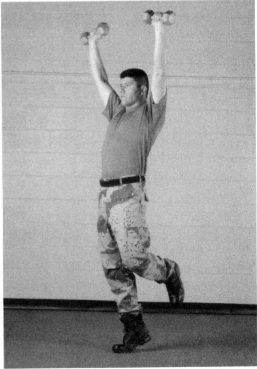

OVERHEAD SQUAT

Start Position: Standing, with dumbbells

Hold dumbbells overhead with a very wide or "snatch" grip. Keeping your arms completely straight and in line with your ears, squat down until your upper thighs are parallel to the floor. Pause for a second before pressing back up with the arms still straight.

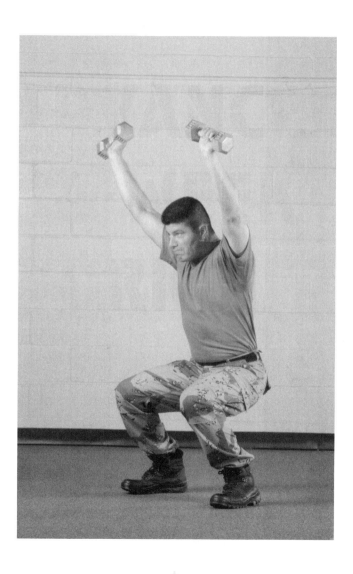

SWISS BALL LEG CURL

Start Position: Lying, with Swiss Ball

Lie on the floor with your feet and lower calves resting on a Swiss ball. With your hands held face down out to the sides, begin by bridging your hips up so that your body forms a diagonal line from your torso to your feet. From there, pull your heels towards your buttocks until the ball is as close to you as possible. Hold momentarily before straightening your legs back out and lowering your hips to the floor.

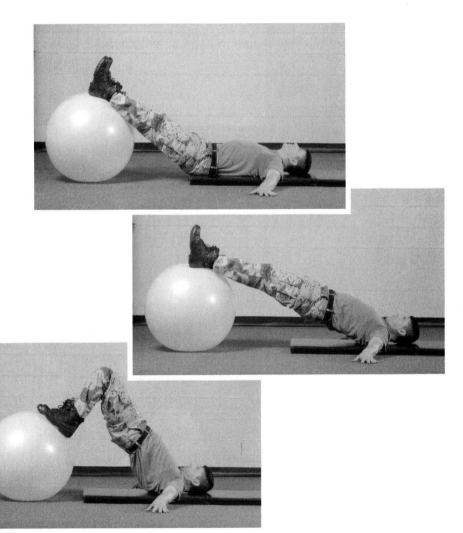

UNILATERAL DEADLIFT

Start Position: Standing, with dumbbells

Stand on one leg and lift the other so the shin is parallel to the floor (like a flamingo). Squat, and try to lightly touch the shin of the non-working leg to the floor. During this exercise, you can allow your upper body to round forward as you are not adding additional stress by doing so. This exercise focuses on the hip gluteus and hamstring muscles.

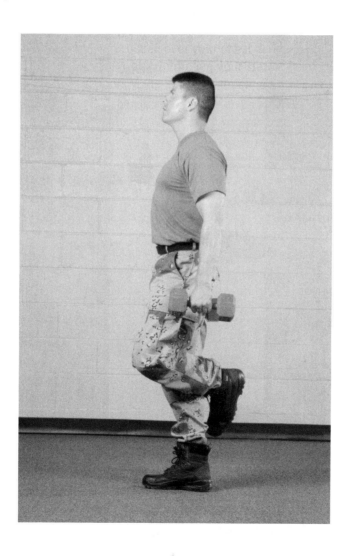

UNILATERAL SQUATS

Start Position: Standing

Lift one leg out in front of you so that your foot is a couple of inches off the floor. Begin by squatting down on the other leg as you allow your torso and arms to come forward as a counter-balance. Squat down as deeply as possible before pressing back up to the start position.

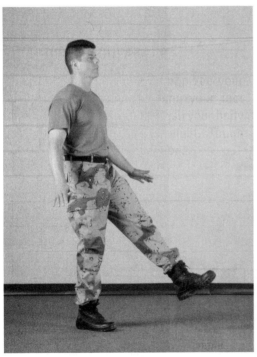 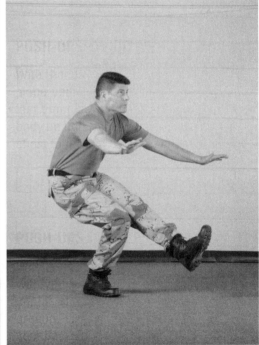

COMBAT DRILLS

Start Position: Standing, in front of exercise mat

Stand up with a padded exercise mat in front of you. Begin by diving down onto the mat so your hands hit first, as you quickly lower yourself into a push-up position. As you begin pushing up, before your arms are completely straight, quickly flip over onto your back. From there use your abs to quickly "roll" up onto your feet and stand up. Turn around, face the net and repeat for the desired number of reps.

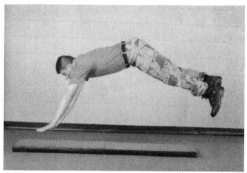

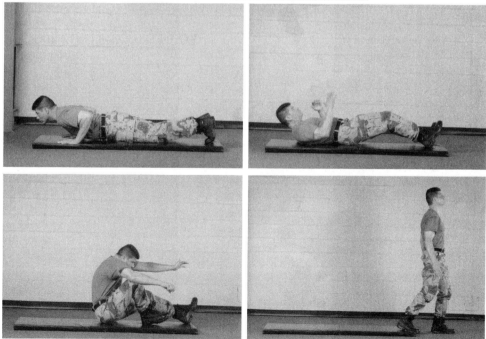

★ ★ ★ ★ ★ ★ ★ ★ ★ ★ ★ ★ ★ ★

ABS/CORE EXERCISES

★ ★ ★ ★ ★ ★ ★ ★ ★ ★ ★ ★ ★ ★

WOODCHOPPER

Start Position: Standing, with medicine ball

Stand with your feet shoulder width apart and your knees slightly bent. Hold the medicine ball with your arms extended. Lift your arms over your right shoulder as you pull your abs into your spine. Quickly and forcefully "chop" the ball down in a sweeping diagonal motion across your body so that you end up with your torso flexed across your thighs and the ball just outside of your left calf. Bring the ball back up in the same sweeping motion, and repeat on the other side.

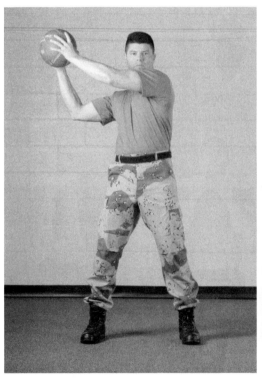 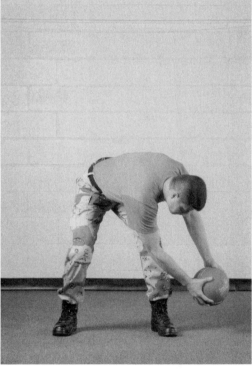

GOOD MORNINGS

Start Position: Standing, with dumbbells on your shoulders

With your feet about shoulder width apart and knees slightly bent, lean forward, breaking at the hips, until your torso is just about parallel to the ground. Pause momentarily before bringing the dumbbells back up to the starting position. Repeat for the desired number of reps.

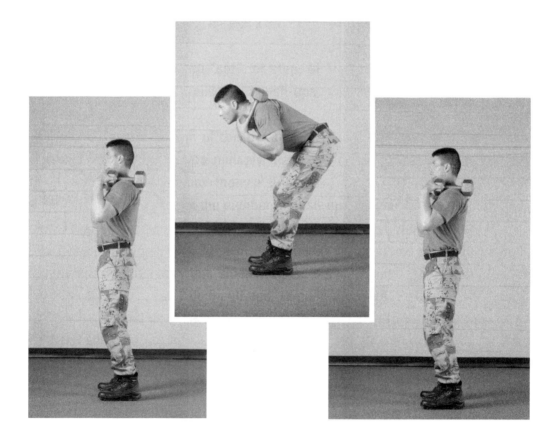

HANGING LEG RAISE

Start Position: Hanging from chin-up bar

Hanging from an overhead bar, use your abdominal muscles and hip flexors to pull your legs up and in toward your chest. Avoid swinging. Exhale at the top of the motion and then slowly lower your legs to the starting position. Repeat for the desired number of reps.

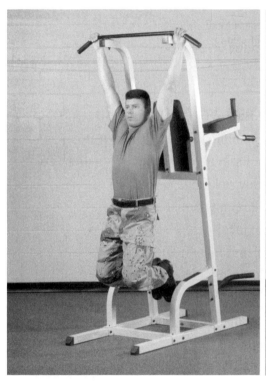
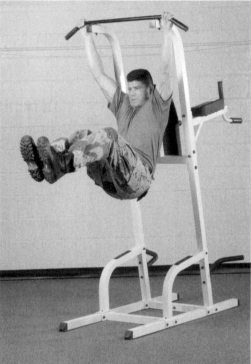

MEDICINE BALL SIT-UPS

Start Position: Lying, with medicine ball

Use a 8- to 10-pound medicine ball for this exercise, depending on your size and strength. Hold the ball with your arms extended over your head. Keeping your arms straight and the ball over your head, sit up until your chest almost touches your thighs. Lower yourself back to the starting position and repeat for the desired number of reps.

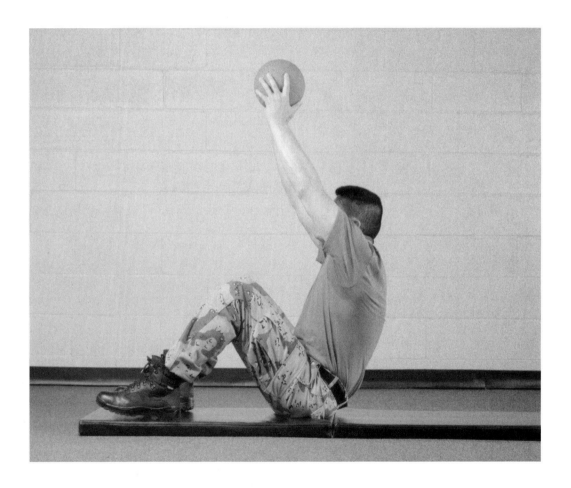

SAXON SIDE BENDS

Start Position: Standing, with dumbbells

With dumbbells, stand with your feet shoulder width apart and knees slightly bent. Straighten your arms over your head so that the weights line up directly over your shoulders. Slowly lean your upper body as far to one side as possible. Once you're leaning over as far as you can, use your abs and oblique muscles to pull yourself back up to the center. Repeat on the other side and then continue for the desired number of reps.

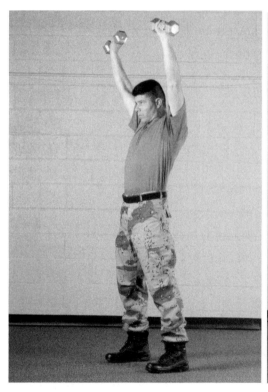
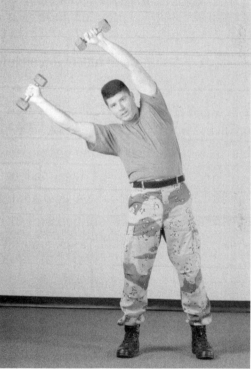

STANDING MEDICINE BALL THROW

Start Position: Standing, with medicine ball

Stand with your feet shoulder width apart and a 6- to 12-pound medicine ball (the weight will depend on your size and strength level) held at arm's length over your head. With your knees slightly bent and arms straight, use your abs to fire the ball into the floor as forcefully as possible about one foot in front of you. In the finish position you should be bent over at the waist so your torso is almost parallel to the floor with your arms extended behind you. The idea is to first use your abs to initiate the downward movement and then use them as brakes to keep you from falling forward. Retrieve the ball and repeat for the desired number of reps.

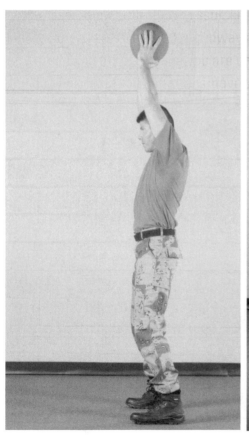 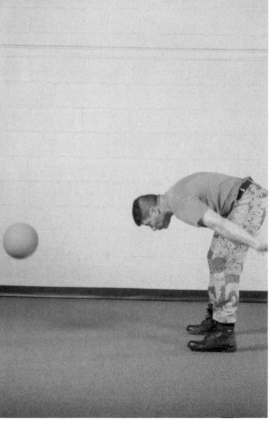

MEDICINE BALL ROTATIONAL THROW

Position: Standing, with medicine ball

Stand with feet shoulder width apart. Hold the ball to one side with your arms extended. Planting your weight, but not tightening your back, turn quickly in the opposite direction and throw the ball. When you throw, don't let your feet come off the floor. Use you core to throw the ball.

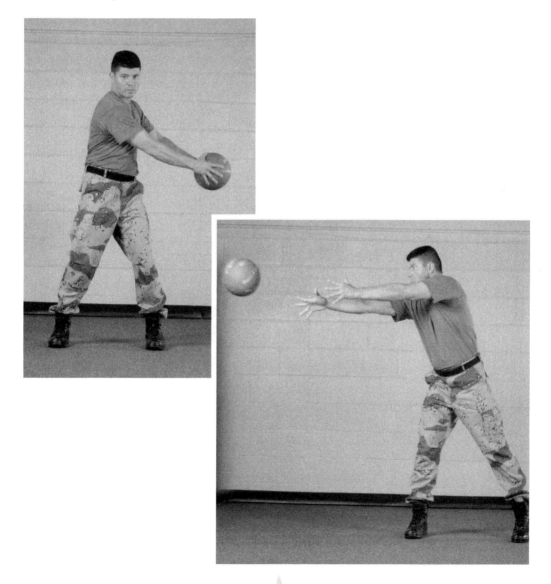

TURKISH GET-UPS

Start Position: Lying, with dumbbell

Start by lying on your back, holding a dumbbell in one hand extended in the air above you; your elbow should be locked. You goal is to stand up while holding the dumbbell without unlocking your elbow and keeping the dumbbell in the air above you.

The first step is usually to turn to your side and prop yourself up on one hand. Next try to get up on one knee. The arm with the dumbbell should still be vertical and locked tight. Now stand up completely. Reverse the movement until you're back at the beginning: lying on the floor with the weight extended above you.

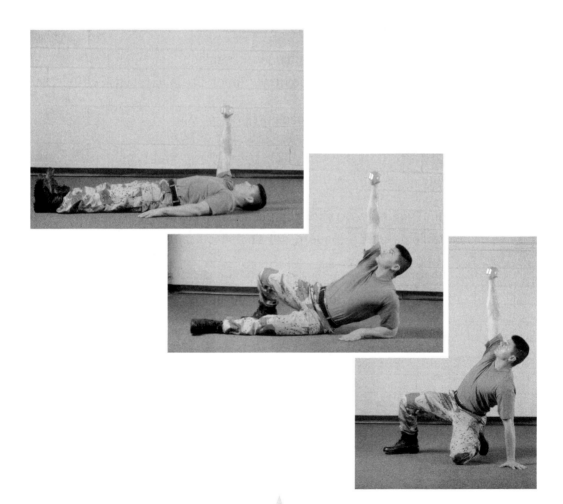

THE
SPECIAL OPS
12-WEEK
WORKOUT
SCHEDULE

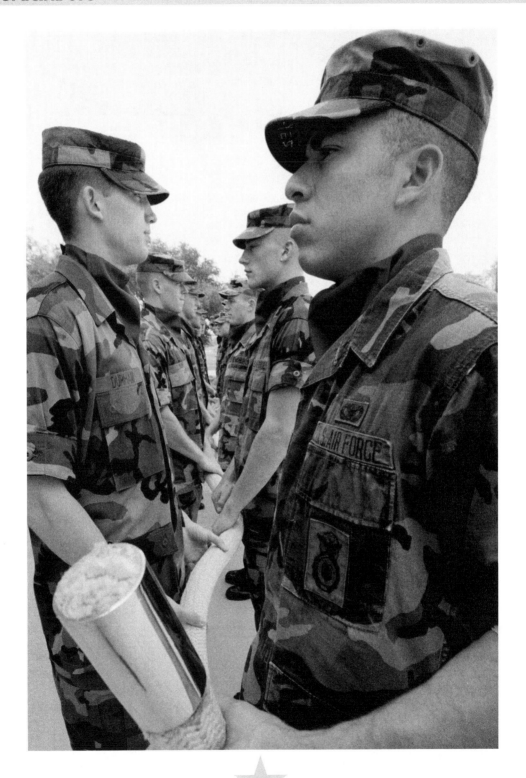

PHASE I: GENERAL PREPARATION

WEEKS 1 THROUGH 4

The goal of this phase is to develop an overall conditioning base, increasing tendon and ligament strength for the more intensive training to follow. Keeping this goal in mind, the workout calls for relatively light resistance and high reps, which will help improve your tolerance to fatigue.

Workout guidelines:

★ This workout is designed as a total-body circuit, to be performed three times per week. Avoid working out three days in a row; the optimal schedule is one day on, one day off (for example, Monday, Wednesday, Friday in week one, Sunday, Tuesday, Thursday in week two).

★ Perform each lift in succession with little to no rest between exercises. This will help optimize the impact of the workout by maintaining a higher level of intensity.

★ After you have completed the last exercise, rest for 60 to 90 seconds before repeating the entire circuit. If you are a beginner, in week 1, complete the circuit twice, adding a third circuit for weeks 3 and 4. For those who are already in good physical shape, start week 1 with three circuits.

★ Each set should consist of 12 to 20 reps, again depending on your starting fitness level. Your goal should be to complete 20 reps of each exercise for each circuit by the end of phase I in week 4.

WEEK 1

MONDAY	WEDNESDAY	FRIDAY

MONDAY

Warm-Up Walk or Jog: 15:00
Stretching: 5:00 to 10:00

Repeat 2 to 3 times:

Dumbbell squat:	12 to 20
3-point push-up:	12 to 20
Unilateral deadlift:	12 to 20
Wide grip pull-up:	12 to 20
Woodchopper:	12 to 20
Low box shuffle:	1:30 to 2:00
Rotational shoulder press:	
12 to 20	
Penta lunge:	12 to 20
Bent-over row:	12 to 20
Overhead balancing calf	
raise:	12 to 20
V-up:	12 to 20
Rest:	::60 to ::90

WEDNESDAY

Warm-Up Walk or Jog: 15:00
Stretching: 5:00 to 10:00

Repeat 2 to 3 times:

Dumbbell squat:	12 to 20
3-point push-up:	12 to 20
Unilateral deadlift:	12 to 20
Wide grip pull-up:	12 to 20
Woodchopper:	12 to 20
Low box shuffle:	1:30 to 2:00
Rotational shoulder press:	
12 to 20	
Penta lunge:	12 to 20
Bent-over row:	12 to 20
Overhead balancing calf	
raise:	12 to 20
V-up:	12 to 20
Rest:	::60 to ::90

FRIDAY

Warm-Up Walk or Jog: 15:00
Stretching: 5:00 to 10:00

Repeat 2 to 3 times:

Dumbbell squat:	12 to 20
3-point push-up:	12 to 20
Unilateral deadlift:	12 to 20
Wide grip pull-up:	12 to 20
Woodchopper:	12 to 20
Low box shuffle:	1:30 to 2:00
Rotational shoulder press:	
12 to 20	
Penta lunge:	12 to 20
Bent-over row:	12 to 20
Overhead balancing calf	
raise:	12 to 20
V-up:	12 to 20
Rest:	::60 to ::90

WEEK 2

SUNDAY

Warm-Up Walk or Jog: 15:00
Stretching: 5:00 to 10:00

Repeat 2 to 3 times:

Dumbbell squat:	12 to 20
3-point push-up:	12 to 20
Unilateral deadlift:	12 to 20
Wide grip pull-up:	12 to 20
Woodchopper:	12 to 20
Low box shuffle:	1:30 to 2:00
Rotational shoulder press:	12 to 20
Penta lunge:	12 to 20
Bent-over row:	12 to 20
Overhead balancing calf raise:	12 to 20
V-up:	12 to 20
Rest:	::60 to ::90

TUESDAY

Warm-Up Walk or Jog: 15:00
Stretching: 5:00 to 10:00

Repeat 2 to 3 times:

Dumbbell squat:	12 to 20
3-point push-up:	12 to 20
Unilateral deadlift:	12 to 20
Wide grip pull-up:	12 to 20
Woodchopper:	12 to 20
Low box shuffle:	1:30 to 2:00
Rotational shoulder press:	12 to 20
Penta lunge:	12 to 20
Bent-over row:	12 to 20
Overhead balancing calf raise:	12 to 20
V-up:	12 to 20
Rest:	::60 to ::90

THURSDAY

Warm-Up Walk or Jog: 15:00
Stretching: 5:00 to 10:00

Repeat 2 to 3 times:

Dumbbell squat:	12 to 20
3-point push-up:	12 to 20
Unilateral deadlift:	12 to 20
Wide grip pull-up:	12 to 20
Woodchopper:	12 to 20
Low box shuffle:	1:30 to 2:00
Rotational shoulder press:	12 to 20
Penta lunge:	12 to 20
Bent-over row:	12 to 20
Overhead balancing calf raise:	12 to 20
V-up:	12 to 20
Rest:	::60 to ::90

WEEK 3

MONDAY		WEDNESDAY		FRIDAY	
Warm-Up Walk or Jog: 15:00		Warm-Up Walk or Jog: 15:00		Warm-Up Walk or Jog: 15:00	
Stretching: 5:00 to 10:00		Stretching: 5:00 to 10:00		Stretching: 5:00 to 10:00	

Repeat 2 to 3 times: (Monday) **Repeat 2 to 3 times:** (Wednesday) **Repeat 2 to 3 times:** (Friday)

Exercise	Monday	Wednesday	Friday
Dumbbell squat:	12 to 20	12 to 20	12 to 20
3-point push-up:	12 to 20	12 to 20	12 to 20
Unilateral deadlift:	12 to 20	12 to 20	12 to 20
Wide grip pull-up:	12 to 20	12 to 20	12 to 20
Woodchopper:	12 to 20	12 to 20	12 to 20
Low box shuffle:	1:30 to 2:00	1:30 to 2:00	1:30 to 2:00
Rotational shoulder press:	12 to 20	12 to 20	12 to 20
Penta lunge:	12 to 20	12 to 20	12 to 20
Bent-over row:	12 to 20	12 to 20	12 to 20
Overhead balancing calf raise:	12 to 20	12 to 20	12 to 20
V-up:	12 to 20	12 to 20	12 to 20
Rest:	::60 to ::90	::60 to ::90	::60 to ::90

WEEK 4

SUNDAY

Warm-Up Walk or Jog: 15:00
Stretching: 5:00 to 10:00

Repeat 2 to 3 times:

Dumbbell squat:	20
3-point push-up:	20
Unilateral deadlift:	20
Wide grip pull-up:	20
Woodchopper:	20
Low box shuffle:	1:30 to 2:00
Rotational shoulder press:	20
Penta lunge:	20
Bent-over row:	20
Overhead balancing calf raise:	20
V-up:	20
Rest:	::60 to ::90

TUESDAY

Warm-Up Walk or Jog: 15:00
Stretching: 5:00 to 10:00

Repeat 2 to 3 times:

Dumbbell squat:	12 to 20
3-point push-up:	12 to 20
Unilateral deadlift:	12 to 20
Wide grip pull-up:	12 to 20
Woodchopper:	12 to 20
Low box shuffle:	1:30 to 2:00
Rotational shoulder press:	12 to 20
Penta lunge:	12 to 20
Bent-over row:	12 to 20
Overhead balancing calf raise:	12 to 20
V-up:	12 to 20
Rest:	::60 to ::90

THURSDAY

Warm-Up Walk or Jog: 15:00
Stretching: 5:00 to 10:00

Repeat 2 to 3 times:

Dumbbell squat:	12 to 20
3-point push-up:	12 to 20
Unilateral deadlift:	12 to 20
Wide grip pull-up:	12 to 20
Woodchopper:	12 to 20
Low box shuffle:	1:30 to 2:00
Rotational shoulder press:	12 to 20
Penta lunge:	12 to 20
Bent-over row:	12 to 20
Overhead balancing calf raise:	12 to 20
V-up:	12 to 20
Rest:	::60 to ::90

PHASE II: MUSCLE GROWTH

WEEKS 5 THROUGH 8

This 4-week phase features one upper and one lower body workout that will be rotated from week to week. You will still work out three times per week, but the emphasis will either be on the upper or lower body. For example, in week one you'll complete two upper body workouts and one lower body workout, and in week two you'll concentrate on the lower body, with two workouts.

While the ultimate goal will still be to increase overall conditioning, this phase features slightly heavier loads and longer rest intervals to stimulate muscle growth.

Workout guidelines:

★ In this phase, reps will range between 8 and 12, with a goal of 12 reps by the end of the four-week period.

★ This workout is conducted using supersets. A superset consists of a set of one exercise immediately followed by a set of another, with no rest in between. While supersets can include many different combinations and numbers of exercises, this workout uses two exercises in each superset. Supersets help raise the intensity of the workout and contribute to faster muscle growth.

★ Complete three supersets, with a 30 to 60 second rest between each. Unlike the previous phase, perform all sets of each group before moving on to the next superset.

WEEK 5

MONDAY

Warm-Up Walk or Jog: 15:00
Stretching: 5:00 to 10:00

Upper Body Workout

Repeat 3 times:
Incline dumbbell press: 8 to 12
Bent-over row: 8 to 12
Rest: ::30 to ::60

Repeat 3 times:
Staggered pull-up: 8 to 12
Pike push-up: 8 to 12
Rest: ::30 to ::60

Repeat 3 times:
Dips: 8 to 12
Hang clean: 8 to 12
Rest: ::30 to ::60

Repeat 3 times:
Hanging leg raise: 8 to 12
Superman: 8 to 12
Rest: ::30 to ::60

WEDNESDAY

Warm-Up Walk or Jog: 15:00
Stretching: 5:00 to 10:00

Lower Body Workout

Repeat 3 times:
Front squat: 8 to 12
Swiss ball leg curl: 8 to 12
Rest: ::30 to ::60

Repeat 3 times:
Lunge: 8 to 12
Superman: 8 to 12
Rest: ::30 to ::60

Repeat 3 times:
Unilateral squat: 8 to 12
Good morning: 8 to 12
Rest: ::30 to ::60

Repeat 3 times:
Saxon side bend: 8 to 12
Flutterkicks: 8 to 12
Rest: ::30 to ::60

FRIDAY

Warm-Up Walk or Jog: 15:00
Stretching: 5:00 to 10:00

Upper Body Workout

Repeat 3 times:
Incline dumbbell press: 8 to 12
Bent-over row: 8 to 12
Rest: ::30 to ::60

Repeat 3 times:
Staggered pull-up: 8 to 12
Pike push-up: 8 to 12
Rest: ::30 to ::60

Repeat 3 times:
Dips: 8 to 12
Hang clean: 8 to 12
Rest: ::30 to ::60

Repeat 3 times:
Hanging leg raise: 8 to 12
Superman: 8 to 12
Rest: ::30 to ::60

WEEK 6

SUNDAY

Warm-Up Walk or Jog: 15:00
Stretching: 5:00 to 10:00

Lower Body Workout

Repeat 3 times:
Front squat: 8 to 12
Swiss ball leg curl: 8 to 12
Rest: ::30 to ::60

Repeat 3 times:
Lunge: 8 to 12
Superman: 8 to 12
Rest: ::30 to ::60

Repeat 3 times:
Unilateral squat: 8 to 12
Good morning: 8 to 12
Rest: ::30 to ::60

Repeat 3 times:
Saxon side bend: 8 to 12
Flutterkicks: 8 to 12
Rest: ::30 to ::60

TUESDAY

Warm-Up Walk or Jog: 15:00
Stretching: 5:00 to 10:00

Upper Body Workout

Repeat 3 times:
Incline dumbbell press: 8 to 12
Bent-over row: 8 to 12
Rest: ::30 to ::60

Repeat 3 times:
Staggered pull-up: 8 to 12
Pike push-up: 8 to 12
Rest: ::30 to ::60

Repeat 3 times:
Dips: 8 to 12
Hang clean: 8 to 12
Rest: ::30 to ::60

Repeat 3 times:
Hanging leg raise: 8 to 12
Superman: 8 to 12
Rest: ::30 to ::60

THURSDAY

Warm-Up Walk or Jog: 15:00
Stretching: 5:00 to 10:00

Lower Body Workout

Repeat 3 times:
Front squat: 8 to 12
Swiss ball leg curl: 8 to 12
Rest: ::30 to ::60

Repeat 3 times:
Lunge: 8 to 12
Superman: 8 to 12
Rest: ::30 to ::60

Repeat 3 times:
Unilateral squat: 8 to 12
Good morning: 8 to 12
Rest: ::30 to ::60

Repeat 3 times:
Saxon side bend: 8 to 12
Flutterkicks: 8 to 12
Rest: ::30 to ::60

WEEK 7

MONDAY

Warm-Up Walk or Jog: 15:00
Stretching: 5:00 to 10:00

Upper Body Workout

Repeat 3 times:
Incline dumbbell press: 8 to 12
Bent-over row: 8 to 12
Rest: ::30 to ::60

Repeat 3 times:
Staggered pull-up: 8 to 12
Pike push-up: 8 to 12
Rest: ::30 to ::60

Repeat 3 times:
Dips: 8 to 12
Hang clean: 8 to 12
Rest: ::30 to ::60

Hanging leg raise: 8 to 12
Superman: 8 to 12
Rest: ::30 to ::60

WEDNESDAY

Warm-Up Walk or Jog: 15:00
Stretching: 5:00 to 10:00

Lower Body Workout

Repeat 3 times:
Front squat: 8 to 12
Swiss ball leg curl: 8 to 12
Rest: ::30 to ::60

Repeat 3 times:
Lunge: 8 to 12
Superman: 8 to 12
Rest: ::30 to ::60

Repeat 3 times:
Unilateral squat: 8 to 12
Good morning: 8 to 12
Rest: ::30 to ::60

Repeat 3 times:
Saxon side bend: 8 to 12
Flutterkicks: 8 to 12
Rest: ::30 to ::60

FRIDAY

Warm-Up Walk or Jog: 15:00
Stretching: 5:00 to 10:00

Upper Body Workout

Repeat 3 times:
Incline dumbbell press: 8 to 12
Bent-over row: 8 to 12
Rest: ::30 to ::60

Repeat 3 times:
Staggered pull-up: 8 to 12
Pike push-up: 8 to 12
Rest: ::30 to ::60

Repeat 3 times:
Dips: 8 to 12
Hang clean: 8 to 12
Rest: ::30 to ::60

Repeat 3 times:
Hanging leg raise: 8 to 12
Superman: 8 to 12
Rest: ::30 to ::60

WEEK 8

SUNDAY	TUESDAY	THURSDAY

Warm-Up Walk or Jog: 15:00
Stretching: 5:00 to 10:00

Lower Body Workout

Repeat 3 times:
Front squat: 12
Swiss ball leg curl: 12
Rest: ::30 to ::60

Repeat 3 times:
Lunge: 12
Superman: 12
Rest: ::30 to ::60

Repeat 3 times:
Unilateral squat: 12
Good morning: 12
Rest: ::30 to ::60

Repeat 3 times:
Saxon side bend: 12
Flutterkicks: 12
Rest: ::30 to ::60

Warm-Up Walk or Jog: 15:00
Stretching: 5:00 to 10:00

Upper Body Workout

Repeat 3 times:
Incline dumbbell press: 12
Bent-over row: 12
Rest: ::30 to ::60

Repeat 3 times:
Staggered pull-up: 12
Pike push-up: 12
Rest: ::30 to ::60

Repeat 3 times:
Dips: 12
Hang clean: 12
Rest: ::30 to ::60

Repeat 3 times:
Hanging leg raise: 12
Superman: 12
Rest: ::30 to ::60

Warm-Up Walk or Jog: 15:00
Stretching: 5:00 to 10:00

Lower Body Workout

Repeat 3 times:
Front squat: 12
Swiss ball leg curl: 12
Rest: ::30 to ::60

Repeat 3 times:
Lunge: 12
Superman: 12
Rest: ::30 to ::60

Repeat 3 times:
Unilateral squat: 12
Good morning: 12
Rest: ::30 to ::60

Repeat 3 times:
Saxon side bend: 12
Flutterkicks: 12
Rest: ::30 to ::60

PHASE III: COMBO TRAINING

WEEKS 9 THROUGH 12

The premise of this phase is to combine plyometric drills with traditional resistance exercises for the ultimate conditioning stimulus. Traditionally, this type of workout calls for a heavy resistance exercise followed by a plyometric one. However, our experience shows that putting the resistance exercise last can increase the results of the workout.

You'll use the same rotating schedule you did in the last phase, but with a slight variation. During the first week you'll perform two plyometric and resistance workouts and one combination lift workout, and then two combination lift workouts and one plyometric and resistance workout in the second week.

WEEK 9

MONDAY	WEDNESDAY	FRIDAY

Warm-Up Walk or Jog: 15:00
Stretching: 5:00 to 10:00
 	
Lunge jump: 6
Overhead squat: 8 to 10
Plyo push-up: 6
Chest press: 8 to 10
Lunge jump: 6
Traveling Lunge: 8 to 10
Standing medicine ball
   throw: 6
Towel pull-up: 8 to 10
Rotational medicine bal
   throw: 6
Medicine ball sit-up: 8 to 10
	Warm-Up Walk or Jog: 15:00
	Stretching: 5:00 to 10:00
	
	The "Bear": 8 to 10
	Front squat: 8 to 10
	Chest press: 8 to 10
	Romanian dead lift and bent-
	   over row: 8 to 10
	Turkish get-up: 8 to 10
	Combat drills: 8 to 10
	Rotational medicine ball
	   throw: 8 to 10
		Warm-Up Walk or Jog: 15:00
		Stretching: 5:00 to 10:00
		
		Lunge jump: 6
		Overhead squat: 8 to 10
		Plyo push-up: 6
		Chest press: 8 to 10
		Lunge jump: 6
		Traveling Lunge: 8 to 10
		Standing medicine ball
		   throw: 6
		Towel pull-up: 8 to 10
		Rotational medicine bal
		   throw: 6
		Medicine ball sit-up: 8 to 10

WEEK 10

SUNDAY

Warm-Up Walk or Jog: 15:00
Stretching: 5:00 to 10:00

The "Bear": 8 to 10
Front squat: 8 to 10
Chest press: 8 to 10
Romanian dead lift and bent-
  over row: 8 to 10
Turkish get-up: 8 to 10
Combat drills: 8 to 10
Rotational medicine ball
  throw: 8 to 10

TUESDAY

Warm-Up Walk or Jog: 15:00
Stretching: 5:00 to 10:00

Lunge jump: 6
Overhead squat: 8 to 10
Plyo push-up: 6
Chest press: 8 to 10
Lunge jump: 6
Traveling Lunge: 8 to 10
Standing medicine ball
  throw: 6
Towel pull-up: 8 to 10
Rotational medicine bal
  throw: 6
Medicine ball sit-up: 8 to 10

THURSDAY

Warm-Up Walk or Jog: 15:00
Stretching: 5:00 to 10:00

The "Bear": 8 to 10
Front squat: 8 to 10
Chest press: 8 to 10
Romanian dead lift and bent-
  over row: 8 to 10
Turkish get-up: 8 to 10
Combat drills: 8 to 10
Rotational medicine ball
  throw: 8 to 10

WEEK 11

MONDAY

Warm-Up Walk or Jog: 15:00
Stretching: 5:00 to 10:00

Lunge jump: 6
Overhead squat: 8 to 10
Plyo push-up: 6
Chest press: 8 to 10
Lunge jump: 6
Traveling Lunge: 8 to 10
Standing medicine ball
  throw: 6
Towel pull-up: 8 to 10
Rotational medicine bal
  throw: 6
Medicine ball sit-up: 8 to 10

WEDNESDAY

Warm-Up Walk or Jog: 15:00
Stretching: 5:00 to 10:00

The "Bear": 8 to 10
Front squat: 8 to 10
Chest press: 8 to 10
Romanian dead lift and bent-
  over row: 8 to 10
Turkish get-up: 8 to 10
Combat drills: 8 to 10
Rotational medicine ball
  throw: 8 to 10

FRIDAY

Warm-Up Walk or Jog: 15:00
Stretching: 5:00 to 10:00

Lunge jump: 6
Overhead squat: 8 to 10
Plyo push-up: 6
Chest press: 8 to 10
Lunge jump: 6
Traveling Lunge: 8 to 10
Standing medicine ball
  throw: 6
Towel pull-up: 8 to 10
Rotational medicine bal
  throw: 6
Medicine ball sit-up: 8 to 10

WEEK 12

SUNDAY

Warm-Up Walk or Jog: 15:00
Stretching: 5:00 to 10:00

The "Bear": 8 to 10
Front squat: 8 to 10
Chest press: 8 to 10
Romanian dead lift and bent-
  over row: 8 to 10
Turkish get-up: 8 to 10
Combat drills: 8 to 10
Rotational medicine ball
  throw: 8 to 10

TUESDAY

Warm-Up Walk or Jog: 15:00
Stretching: 5:00 to 10:00

Lunge jump: 6
Overhead squat: 8 to 10
Plyo push-up: 6
Chest press: 8 to 10
Lunge jump: 6
Traveling Lunge: 8 to 10
Standing medicine ball
  throw: 6
Towel pull-up: 8 to 10
Rotational medicine bal
  throw: 6
Medicine ball sit-up: 8 to 10

THURSDAY

Warm-Up Walk or Jog: 15:00
Stretching: 5:00 to 10:00

The "Bear": 8 to 10
Front squat: 8 to 10
Chest press: 8 to 10
Romanian dead lift and bent-
  over row: 8 to 10
Turkish get-up: 8 to 10
Combat drills: 8 to 10
Rotational medicine ball
  throw: 8 to 10

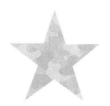

PART III:

ADVANCED 6-WEEK WORKOUTS

WORKOUT NOTES

The following workouts are advanced programs and *not* intended for beginners. They are designed to prepare you for any one of the Special Operations Command Units: Navy SEALs, Air Force PJ / CCT, Army Special Forces—the Special Forces Assessment and Selection (SFAS), Qualification Course as well as RIP, Ranger Indoctrination Program (Green Berets and Ranger School). The previous 12-week programs are to be used to build a base of torso strength and proper muscular development IF you have never attempted such challenging routines as Ruck Marches, swimming with fins in open ocean, and hundreds of repetitions of push-ups, sit-ups, and pull-ups.

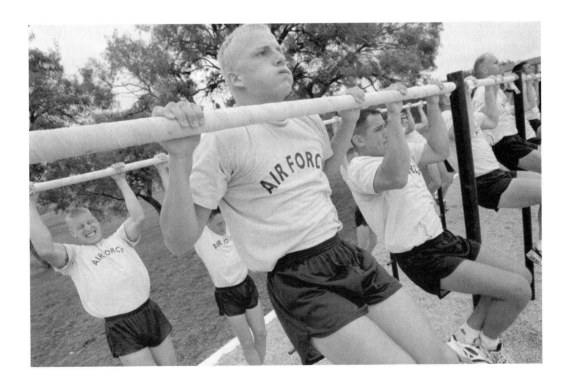

KEY EXERCISES: SIT-UPS & FLUTTER KICKS

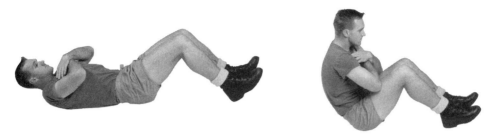

SIT-UPS: REGULAR

Lay on your back with your arms crossed over your chest and your knees slightly bent. Raise your upper body off the floor by contracting your stomach muscles. Touch your elbows to your thighs and repeat. Make sure you touch your shoulder blades to the floor each time.

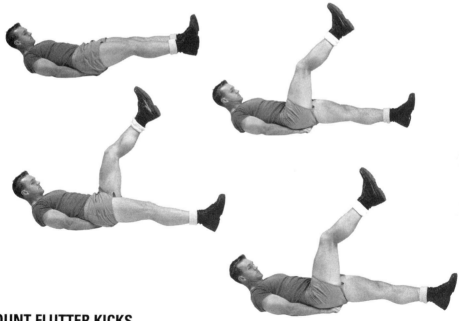

4-COUNT FLUTTER KICKS

Place your hands under your hips. Lift legs 6 inches off the ground and begin "walking," raising each leg approximately 3 feet off the ground. Keep your legs straight and constantly moving. With each "step" you take, count 1, so the sequence will go as follows: 1, 2, 3, 1; 1, 2, 3, 2; 1, 2, 3, 3; . . . for the specified number of repetitions.

KEY EXERCISES: PUSH-UPS

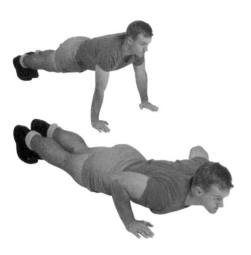

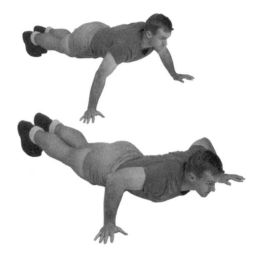

PUSH-UPS: REGULAR

With hands at shoulder width, place your palms on the ground, keeping your feet together and back straight. Push your body up until your arms are straight. Touch chest to ground each repetition.

PUSH-UPS: WIDE

With hands wider than shoulder width, place your palms on the ground, keeping feet together and back straight. Push your body up until your arms are straight. Touch chest to ground each repetition.

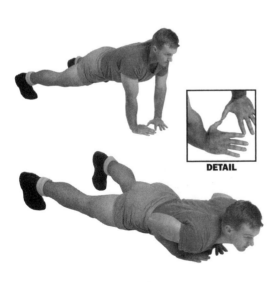

DETAIL

PUSH-UPS: TRICEPS

With hands touching, forming a triangle with your index fingers and thumbs meeting (as shown above), place palms on the ground, spreading your legs and keeping your back straight. Push your body up until your arms are straight. Touch chest to hands each repetition.

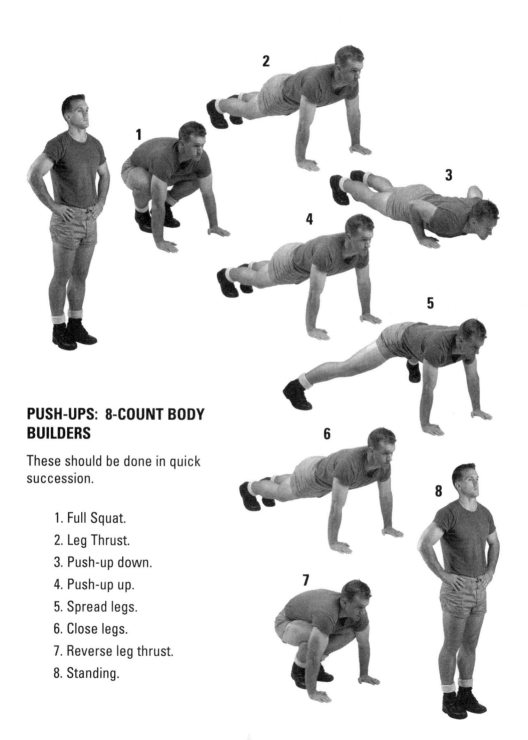

PUSH-UPS: 8-COUNT BODY BUILDERS

These should be done in quick succession.

1. Full Squat.
2. Leg Thrust.
3. Push-up down.
4. Push-up up.
5. Spread legs.
6. Close legs.
7. Reverse leg thrust.
8. Standing.

KEY EXERCISES: PULL-UPS

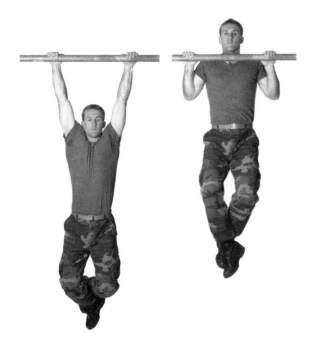

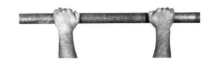

REGULAR GRIP

With hands at shoulder width (see below), grab the bar and pull yourself up so your chin is lifted above the bar. Hold yourself above the bar for one second and let yourself down in a slow, controlled manner.

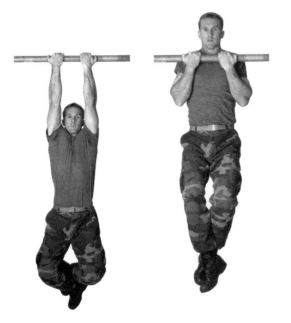

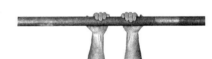

REVERSE GRIP

With your palms facing you (see below), grab the bar and pull your chin over the bar. Complete specified number of repetitions.

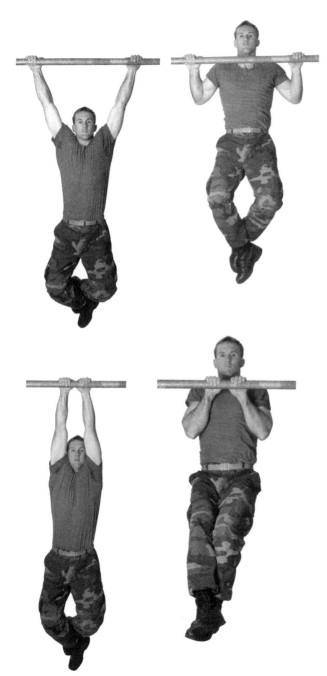

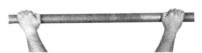

WIDE GRIP

With hands wider than shoulder width, and palms facing away from you (see below), grab the bar and pull your chin above it. Complete specified number of repetitions.

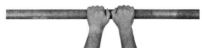

CLOSE GRIP

With your hands touching (or within 1 inch of each other), and palms facing away from you (see below), grab the bar and pull your chin over the bar. Complete specified number of repetitions.

PYRAMID WORKOUTS

If you take a look at one of the pyramids, you will notice that it is numbered on both sides. It goes from 1 to 10 on one side, and then 10 to 1 on the other. Each number represents a step in the pyramid. Your goal is to climb the pyramid all the way up and then all the way back down. So, you can consider each step a "set" of your workout.

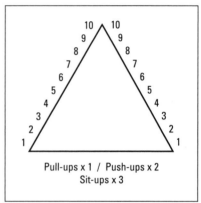

Pull-ups x 1 / Push-ups x 2
Sit-ups x 3

At the bottom, you will see:
pull-ups x 1, push-ups x 2, sit-ups x 3

This means that at *each* "set", or step, of the pyramid, you perform 1 pull-up , 2 push-ups, and 3 sit-ups.

You start at the bottom of the pyramid, at number 1. For each set, you multiply that set number by 1; that tells you how many pull-ups to do. You multiply it by 2 to get the number of push-ups, and multiply by 3 for sit-ups. You keep progressing until you get to the top of the pyramid, or your max. At step 10 you perform 10 pull-ups, 20 push-ups, and 30 sit-ups. Now you start working your way back down the other side. The next set you do will be at step 9 on the way back down. So, you'll do 9 pull-ups, 18 push-ups, and 27 sit-ups. Keep going until you've worked all the way back down to step 1. Here is a number summary of the pyramid:

Going up the pyramid (or half pyramid workout):

Set 1	1 pull-up	2 push-ups	3 sit-ups
Set 2	2 pull-ups	4 push-ups	6 sit-ups
Set 3	3 pull-ups	6 push-ups	9 sit-ups
Set 4	4 pull-ups	8 push-ups	12 sit-ups
Set 5	5 pull-ups	10 push-ups	15 sit-ups

(Your first sets are basically a warm-up)

Set 6	6 pull-ups	12 push-ups	18 sit-ups
Set 7	7 pull-ups	14 push-ups	21 sit-ups
Set 8	8 pull-ups	16 push-ups	24 sit-ups
Set 9	9 pull-ups	18 push-ups	27 sit-ups
Set 10	10 pull-ups	20 push-ups	30 sit-ups

(Here is where you should fail / max out)

Go down the pyramid: (or reverse order pyramid = toughest to easiest number of reps.

SWIM WORKOUTS

Note: *Do not do these workouts by yourself. In fact, never swim underwater alone or without a lifeguard.*

HYPOXIC PYRAMID (STROKES PER BREATH)

This workout makes ordinary swimming seem easy and will actually help make your swimming, running, and overall endurance. By not allowing yourself to breathe as often as you would like, you are training like someone in higher altitudes. Therefore, when you test yourself and breathe regularly, you will be like the high altitude athlete going to sea-level to compete.

This particular workout gets increasingly difficult after each 100m you swim. By adding 2 strokes to your breathing pattern every 100m, you will find the need to breathe more demanding. Simply climb the pyramid, making each set of 100m a step. At each step you will add two more strokes per breath. You will be breathing less per length on every step up the pyramid until you reach the maximum of 10 strokes per breath. A stroke is each arm pull, so the count would be this for a 4 strokes per breath step on the pyramid: 1, 2, 3, 4, breathe. This translates to left arm pull, right arm pull, left arm pull, right arm pull, breathe.

If you hold your breath for at least half of the stroke count and then start exhaling slowly, you can make it through the pyramid with little difficulty. It does take time before you can do this workout with no rest at all. So for the first few times, take 20 to 30 seconds rest if you need to between steps of the pyramid.

HYPOXIC PYRAMID (STROKES PER LENGTH)

This hypoxic workout requires you to swim a known distance with a certain number of breaths. For instance, you will swim 50 meters breathing only 4 times, then 3 times, then 2 times, then only 1 time, for a total of 200 meters. Try this workout several more times for a total of 1000 meters.

SWIM PT

This is a great way to squeeze swimming and upper body PT into the same workout. Simply swim the specified distances (usually 100 yards or meters), get out of the pool and do push-ups, abdominal exercises, and pull-ups. Repeat this sequence at least 10 times.

SIDE STROKE WITH FINS

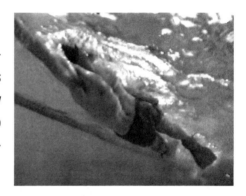

This is one of the best leg workouts available. Your hamstrings, hip flexors, and ankles will become strong and ripped after a few months of swimming with fins. It is similar to the side stroke without fins with only the following differences:

Constant flutterkicks. With fins on your feet, your biggest source of power will naturally be your legs, so kick constantly in order to be propelled through the water.

Constant flutterkicks and glide position. Breathe as the bottom arm pulls toward your body. Recover both arms over your head together with a forceful kick and hold for 2 to 3 seconds as you glide in the streamlined position.

Open water: Swimming in straight line. Every five or so strokes, it is important to look forward to check whether or not you are swimming in a straight line. This does not need to be done in the swimming pool; however, it is important in the open ocean to have a visual reference when surface swimming to check accuracy.

Sample Workout with Fins:

Swim with fins: 500 yards with fins and 500 without fins using the stroke of your choice.

COMBAT SWIMMER STROKE (CSS)

The CSS, an updated version of the traditional sidestroke, is a relaxing and super efficient swim stroke. Whether you are a beginning swimmer or an aspiring Navy SEAL, Army SF, or Air Force PJ, this stroke can help you efficiently move through the water.

When you find yourself in deep water with a lot of distance to cover, the CSS will serve you well especially when you are wearing fins. You will tire less quickly if you learn to perform this stroke properly.

Here's the Combat Swimmer Stroke, broken down into four parts:

Kick off the Wall. The object of the CSS and side stroke is efficiency: You should try to get across a 25m pool in as few strokes as possible. If you are doing more than 10 strokes per length you are working too hard. In fact, the fastest and best swimmers get across a 25m pool in 3 to 5 strokes.

The Start: In a big squat position against the wall, push off and stay as streamlined as possible as you glide at least 5 to 10 yards off the wall. Place your hands on top of each other, place your bicep on your ears, and lock out your arms, streamlined positioning like a rocket.

The Glide. With a big double arm pull, add the other 3 to 5 yards to your glide by pulling with your back and biceps and pushing water with your arms using your triceps.

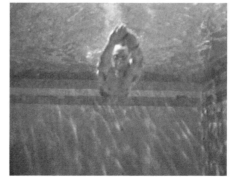

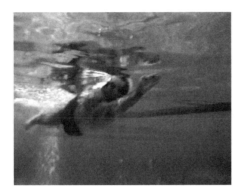

Arm Motion. After the arm pull, it is time to breathe. Twist and breathe then start using the top arm pull as shown. Both arms recover together forward, but the top arm pulls from overhead all the way to your hips (like freestyle stroke). Then the bottom arm pulls a half stroke (like breast stroke) and both arms recover together. Breathe as the top arm completes its pull and the bottom arm begins its pull.

Scissor Kick. Use the scissor kick and time your kicks so your top leg always goes forward (no matter what side you are on). You should kick just after both arms have pulled and are recovering, adding more glide to each stroke.

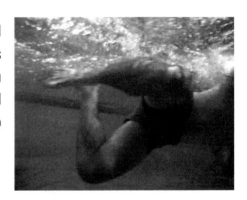

SWIM DRILLS FOR SEAL AND PJS

These drills are for you to practice prior to PJ and SEAL training. Do NOT practice tying your hands behind your back and your feet together and getting into the pool as in the drown-proofing test.

Tread water. Using arms and legs relax and tread water. Try it without your hands, lifting your hands out of the water for 5 minutes

Bottom bounce. With hands behind you and feet together, bounce off the bottom 20 times.

Float. Keep hands and feet in same position and bend 90 degrees at the waist and float for 10 to 20 breaths.

Swim 50 to 100 yards with feet and hands in the same position as above. Use the dolphin kick.

Frontward and backward flips in the water with hands and feet as above.

Pick up goggles or face mask with your teeth at the bottom of the pool.

Snorkel buddy breathing. Practice taking a snorkel in and out of your mouth while breathing near the surface. This is a challenging test at PJ school and BUDS.

Sequence of events for Swim Drills:
Total Time: 10 minutes
Tread water: 5:00
Bottom bounce: 1:00
Float: 1:00
Swim: 100 meters
Front/back flip
Pick up goggles

★ STEW SMITH'S RUCKING TIPS ★

Before starting the rucking workouts, keep these pointers in mind.

- For forced marches, select boots that are comfortable and well broken-in (not worn out).

- Wear lightweight fatigues and thick socks (not new socks). Army issue boots are excellent if fitted properly.

- Use map and compass techniques whenever possible during forced march cross-country workouts.

- Insoles specifically designed to absorb shock will reduce the chance of injury.

- Practice proper rucksack marching and walking technique:

- Weight of the body must be kept directly over the feet, and the sole of the shoe must be flat on the ground, taking small steps at a steady pace.

- Knees must be locked on every step to rest muscles of the legs (especially when going uphill).

- When walking cross-country, step over and around obstacles—never step on them.

- When traveling up steep slopes, keep the back straight and knees bent to take up shock of each step.

- When descending steep slopes, keep the back straight and knees bent to take up shock of each step. Dig in heels on each step.

- Practice walking as fast as you can with rucksack. Do not run with rucksack. When testing, you may have to trot to maintain time, but try not to do this during training; it may injure you.

- A good rucksack pace is accomplished by continuous movement with short breaks (5 minutes) every 6 to 8 miles.

- If you cannot ruckmarch, do squats with your rucksack: 5 sets of 100 reps or until muscles fatigue.

- On each day (not listed in training program), conduct less strenuous workouts such as biking and short or slow runs. To complement push-up workouts, weight-lifting exercises should be included (for development of upper-body strength) in easy day workout schedule. Swim as often as you can (500 meters or more).

- Once a high level of physical fitness is attained, a maintenance workout program should be applied using the hard and easy workout concept. Once in shape, stay in shape. Do not stop this program. If you have meet all the goals, then modify program by increasing distance and weight and decreasing times. Be smart. Don't injure yourself.

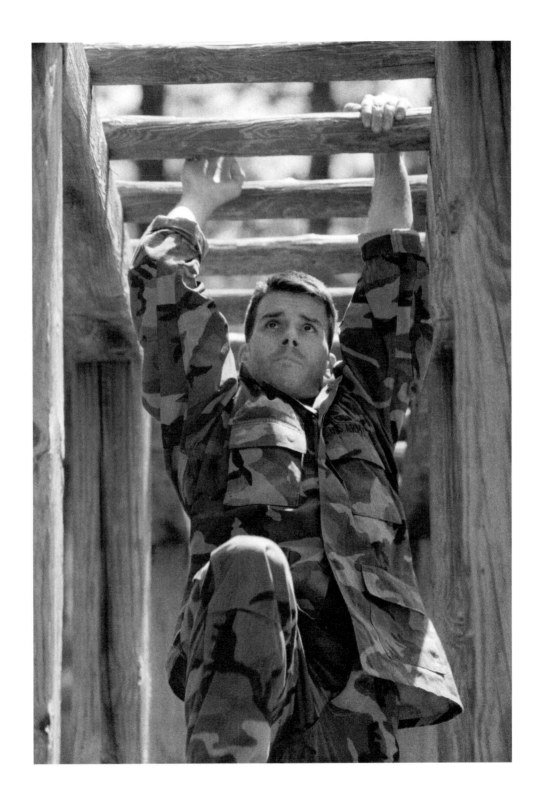

★ ARMY RANGER & GREEN BERET WORKOUT

WEEK 1 ARMY RANGER & GREEN BERET WORKOUT

MONDAY

Warm-Up and Stretch: 5:00

Army PFT

Max push-ups
Max sit-ups
Max pull-ups (extra)
Rest 10:00
2-mile run

Must score 240 minimum by
end of SFAS
And a score of 206 to enter

Swim PT

Swim 500m timed
Swim 50m in uniform

TUESDAY

Warm-Up and Stretch: 5:00

3-mile run timed

Repeat 10 times:
  Jumping Jacks   10
  Squats   20

PT

Repeat 5 times:
  Towel pull-ups: 10
  Weighted squats: 20
  Woodchoppers: 20
  Traveling lunges: 20
  Overhead squats: 10

Abs

Repeat 2 times:
  Sit-ups: 50
  Windshield wipers: 25
  Flutterkicks: 25
  Side bends: 20

Ruck

4 miles in 60:00 or less

WEDNESDAY

Warm-Up, Run, Stretch: 5:00

Upperbody Weight / PT Circuit

Repeat 2 times (no rest):
  Dips: max + 3 negatives
  Max sit-ups in 1:00
  Max bench press
  Max push-ups in 1:00
  Max flutterkicks in 1:00
  Max military press (light
    weight)
  Bent over rows: 30 reps/arm
  Max leg levers in 1:00
  Supermans: 1:00

Swim PT

Swim 500m

A NOTE ABOUT NUTRITION

The *Army Ranger & Green Beret Workout* is designed to build muscle, speed and endurance and to prepare you for Special Ops training. It's important to note that food intake is seriously limited to 1 to 2 meals a day and ruck marches span 15 to 20 miles in a day; that means you will lose significant amounts of weight in both muscle and fat. Some people have lost 20 to 30 pounds through the course. So you should bulk up prior to going if you are naturally lean. Do not bulk up so much that it impacts your fitness level, but remember that adding a few pounds will not hurt you.

ARMY RANGER & GREEN BERET WORKOUT   WEEK 1

THURSDAY

Warm-Up and Stretch: 5:00

Ruck

8 miles with 40lbs

Back & Legs

Repeat 2 to 3 times:
Squats:	30
Regular pull-ups:	10
Reverse pull-ups:	10

Supersets

Repeat 3 times:
Overhead squats:	10
Lunges:	30
Calves:	25

Back / Biceps

Repeat 2 times:
Pull-ups:	max
Bent over rows:	20
Side bends:	20

FRIDAY

Warm-Up and Stretch: 5:00

Run / PT / Run

Run:	1 mile
Crunches:	100
Push-ups:	75
Run:	1 mile
Sit-ups:	75
Push-ups:	65
Run:	1 mile
Sit-ups:	50
Push-ups:	50

Pull-ups: 3 times max
Rope climbs: 3 (or do pull-ups with a towel for the grip)

SATURDAY

Warm-Up and Stretch: 5:00

Ruck / Swim / Run

Ruck: 8 miles in 2 hours
Swim: 500yd timed
Repeat swim: Total 1000yd +
50m BDU swim
Run: 4 miles timed

WEEK 2   ARMY RANGER & GREEN BERET WORKOUT

MONDAY

Warm-Up and Stretch: 5:00

PT

Repeat 5 times:
Pull-ups:	max
Bench press:	10
or push-ups:	20
Abs of choice:	50

Repeat 5 times:
Push-ups:	20
Pull-ups:	
wide grip:	10
regular grip:	10
reverse grip:	10
Sit-ups:	50

Run

5-mile track workout:
Run 2 miles timed
1-mile sprint / 1/2 mile jog
1-mile sprint / 1/2 mile jog

TUESDAY

Jog 5:00 / Stretch legs

PT

Repeat 5 times:
Bike or run (fast):	5:00
Lunges (each leg):	30
Abs of choice:	100
Squats:	30

Ruck

10-mile timed ruck under
3 hours with 35 lbs

WEDNESDAY

Warm-Up and Stretch: 5:00

Upperbody PT / Abs

Repeat 10 times:
Push-ups:	10
Jumping jacks:	20

Repeat 5 times:
Bench press:	20
Crunches:	50
Wide push-ups:	10
Regular push-ups:	10
Triceps push-ups:	10
Abs of choice:	50

Swim 500m times 2

ARMY RANGER & GREEN BERET WORKOUT   WEEK 2

THURSDAY

Warm-Up and Stretch: 5:00

Ruck/PT

10-mile ruck
At every mile, stop and do
20 squats with ruck on

Run 4 miles at 7:00 to 8:00
pace

FRIDAY

Warm-Up and Stretch: 5:00

Upperbody PT

Repeat 5 times:
  Bench press: 20, 15, 10
  reps; increasing weight,
  nonstop

or

Repeat 5 times:
  Push-ups: 40
  Reg crunches: 25
  Sit-ups: 25
  Push-ups: 20
  Flutterkicks: 50
  Towel pull-ups: max
  Rope climbs times 3
  (optional)

Lower Back Exercise

Supermans: 1:00

Run

2-mile sprint

SATURDAY

Warm-Up and Stretch: 5:00

Mini Triathlon

Run: 5 miles in 40:00
Swim: 1000m CSS
Bike: 60:00 or 4-mile ruck

WEEK 3 ARMY RANGER & GREEN BERET WORKOUT

MONDAY

Warm-Up and Stretch: 5:00

Army PFT

Max push-ups in 2:00
Max sit-ups in 2:00
Max Army run: 2 miles

Run, bike, or swim: 30:00

TUESDAY

Warm-Up and Stretch: 5:00

Lower Body Day

Bike or Run
Repeat 4 times:
  Sprint 1/2 mile or bike
    1 mile
  Max squats in 1:00
  Lunges: 15 / leg
  Max crunches in 1:00

Ruck

12-mile Ruck March with
  40 lbs

Stretch

Stretch head to toe

WEDNESDAY

Warm-Up and Stretch: 5:00

Pull-Up PT

Pull-Up Pyramid (see
  page 114)

Rest with 25 sit-ups or
crunches between each pull-
up set.

Run or bike 20:00

Ruck

1 hour

ARMY RANGER & GREEN BERET WORKOUT   WEEK 3

THURSDAY

Warm-Up and Stretch: 5:00

Rest Day

FRIDAY

Warm-Up and Stretch: 5:00

Run

2-mile run timed

Ruck

6-mile Ruck March

PT

Repeat 2 times:

Pull-ups:	10
Crunches:	50
Pull-ups:	max
Medicine ball sit-ups:	25
Pull-ups:	max − 1
Crunches:	50
Pull-ups:	max − 2
Flutterkicks:	25
Pull-ups:	max − 3
Sit-ups:	25
Pull-ups:	max − 4
Stomach stretch:	1:00
Supermans:	1:00

SATURDAY

Warm-Up and Stretch: 5:00

Pyramid to Failure

Push-ups times 3
Abs times 5
Dips times 3

See page 114. Start at bottom, go to max sets in all events, and then back to the bottom. If you fail in one event, dips for example, before the others, just do negatives or assisteds until you max on two of the three events.

Run or Bike

Your choice:
  2-mile run
    or 5-mile bike timed

Ruck

5-mile, 35 lb Ruck March

WEEK 4   ARMY RANGER & GREEN BERET WORKOUT

MONDAY

Warm-Up and Stretch: 5:00

PT / Circuit

Repeat 5 times:
Jumping jacks:	20
Push-ups:	20
Squats w/heel raise:	30

Repeat 5 times:
Jumping jacks:	20
Pike push-ups:	20
Lunges:	20/leg

Repeat 5 times:
Jumping jacks:	20
Triceps push-ups:	10
Pull-ups:	max

Repeat 5 times:
Abs of choice:	50
Lower back:	::20
Wide push-ups:	20

Swim / Jog / Ruck: 30:00 each

TUESDAY

Warm-Up and Stretch: 5:00

Run

3-Mile Track Workout:

Three sets of:
Sprint:	1/4 mile
Jog:	1/4 mile

Six sets of:
Sprint:	1/8 mile
Jog:	1/8 mile

Ruck

4 miles with 35 lbs

PT

Repeat 4 times:
Sit-ups:	50
L/R sit-ups:	25 each side
Flutterkicks:	50
Leg levers:	50
Side bends:	20
Supermans:	1:00

WEDNESDAY

Warm-Up and Stretch: 5:00

PT with Clock

(Note: Pace the sit-ups, not the push-ups)
Max pull-ups
Max push-ups in 2:00
Max sit-ups in 2:00
Rest 2:00
Max pull-ups
50 to 60 sit-ups in 1:00
Max push-ups in 1:00
Rest 2:00
Max pull-ups
25 to 30 sit-ups in ::30
Max push-ups in ::30
Rest 2:00
Max pull-ups
10 to 15 sit-ups in ::15
Max push-ups in ::15

Run / PT

Repeat 8 times:

Sprint 1/4 mile
Push-ups: 10
Abs of choice: 20

ARMY RANGER & GREEN BERET WORKOUT   WEEK 4

THURSDAY

Warm-Up and Stretch: 5:00

Ruck

14-mile ruck with 50 lbs

500m swim

FRIDAY

Warm-Up and Stretch: 5:00

Push-up/Crunch Superset

10 cycles of:
Regular push-ups:	10
Crunches:	10
Wide push-ups:	10
Sit-ups:	10
Triceps push-ups:	10
Flutterkicks:	20

Run

4-Mile Track Workout
Jog 1 mile in 8:00

3 sets of:
Sprint:	1/4 mile
Jog:	1/4 mile

6 sets of:
Sprint:	1/8 mile
Jog:	1/8 mile

Cooldown swim if available:
Swim with cammies 100m
then 500m without.

SATURDAY

Warm-Up and Stretch: 5:00

Repeat 3 times:
  Wide pull-ups: 2, 4, 6, 8
  Regular pull-ups: 2, 4, 6, 8
  Reverse pull-ups: 2, 4, 6, 8

6-mile run timed

WEEK 5 ARMY RANGER & GREEN BERET WORKOUT

MONDAY

Warm-Up and Stretch: 5:00

Push-up/Crunch Superset

(20:00 workout)
Repeat 10 times:
Regular push-ups:	10
Crunches:	10
Wide push-ups:	10
Sit-ups:	10
Triceps push-ups:	10
Flutterkicks:	20

Pull-ups

Wide pull-ups: 2, 4, 6, 8, 10
Regular pull-ups: 2, 4, 6, 8, 10
Reverse pull-ups: 2, 4, 6, 8, 10
Towel pull-ups: 2, 4, 6, 8, 10

Run

4-Mile Track Workout
Jog 1 mile in 8:00

Three sets of:
Sprint:	1/4 mile
Jog:	1/4 mile

Six sets of:
Sprint:	1/8 mile
Jog:	1/8 mile

TUESDAY

Warm-Up and Stretch: 5:00

Run

6 miles at 7:00 to 8:00 pace

Swim

Swim 500m

Stretch

Total body stretch

WEDNESDAY

Warm-Up and Stretch: 5:00

Run

4-mile timed run

Swim / PT Set

Repeat 10 times:
Swim:	100m
Push-ups:	20
Abs of choice:	20

PT

Repeat 3 times:
Pull-ups:	max
Rope climbs:	3

(Use towel hung over the bar as a grip for rope simulation.)

ARMY RANGER & GREEN BERET WORKOUT   WEEK 5

THURSDAY

Warm-Up and Stretch: 5:00

Rest Day

FRIDAY

Warm-Up and Stretch: 5:00

PT with the Clock

(Note: Pace the sit-ups, not the push-ups.)

Max pull-ups
Max push-ups in 2:00
Max sit-ups in 2:00
Rest 2:00
Max pull-ups
50 to 60 sit-ups in 1:00
Max push-ups in 1:00
Rest 2:00
Max pull-ups
25 to 30 sit-ups in ::30
Max push-ups in ::30
Rest 2:00
Max pull-ups
10 to 15 sit-ups in ::15
Max push-ups in ::15

SATURDAY

Warm-Up and Stretch: 5:00

Ruck

14-mile ruck with 50 lbs

Swim

500m swim

Stretch

Total body stretch

SUNDAY

Leg PT / Run

6-mile timed run
Every mile, stop and do:
   30 squats
   30 lunges

WEEK 6   ARMY RANGER & GREEN BERET WORKOUT

MONDAY	TUESDAY	WEDNESDAY
Warm-Up and Stretch: 5:00	Warm-Up and Stretch: 5:00	Warm-Up and Stretch: 5:00

MONDAY

Warm-Up and Stretch: 5:00

Rest Day

TUESDAY

Warm-Up and Stretch: 5:00

Army PFT
Max push-ups
Max sit-ups in 2:00
Army run: 2 miles

Cardio
Run, bike, or swim: 30:00

WEDNESDAY

Warm-Up and Stretch: 5:00

Ruck
5-mile ruck with 50 lbs
    Every mile, stop and do:
    30 squats with ruck on

ARMY RANGER & GREEN BERET WORKOUT   WEEK 6

THURSDAY	FRIDAY	SATURDAY

Warm-Up and Stretch: 5:00

Swim

Swim 500 to 1000m

Warm-Up and Stretch: 5:00

Push-up / Crunch Superset

Repeat 10 times in 20:00:

Regular push-ups:	10
Crunches:	10
Wide push-ups:	10
Sit-ups:	10
Triceps push-up:	10
Flutterkicks:	20

Swim / PT

Repeat 10 times:

CSS (see page 117):	100m
Push-ups:	20
Sit-ups:	20

Warm-Up and Stretch: 5:00

Ruck

This is the Green Beret assessment test.

Ruck 18 miles with 50 lbs
   at least 4.5 hours on road <u>or</u>
   6 hours cross-country

Swim

500m swim

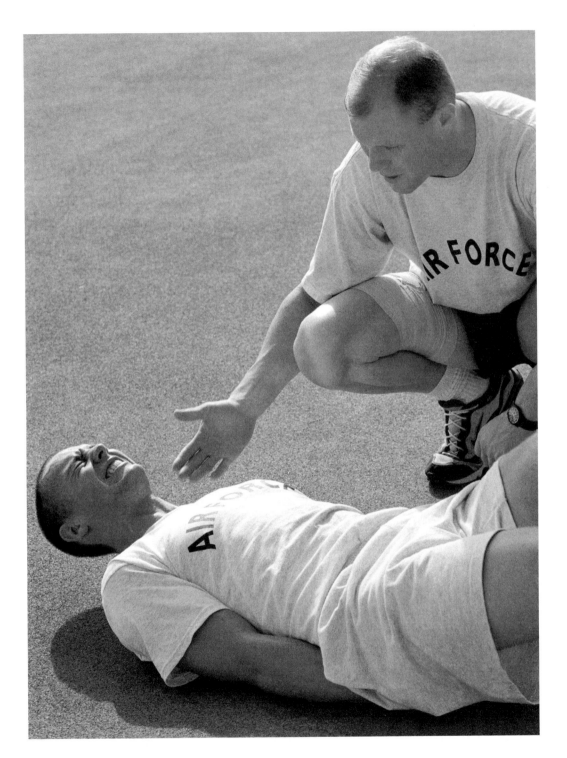

★ AIR FORCE PJ/CCT WORKOUT

WEEK 1   AIR FORCE PJ/CCT WORKOUT

MONDAY

Warm-Up and Stretch: 5:00

PJ/CCT Test

Timed 500-yard CSS
Max flutterkicks in 2:00
Max push-ups in 2:00
Rest 2:00
Max sit-ups or crunches in 2:00
Rest: 2:00
Max pull-ups:
1.5-mile sprint

Pool drills to work on technique: 20:00

TUESDAY

Warm-Up and Stretch: 5:00

Lower Body PT

Repeat 4 times:
  Sprint: 1 mile
  Max squats in 1:00
  Max calves in 1:00
  Lunges: 25/leg
  Max sit-ups or crunches in 2:00

WEDNESDAY

Warm-Up and Stretch: 5:00

Swim Test Day

500-yard CSS
Rest and stretch: 5:00
500-yard freestyle

PT

Max push-ups in 2:00
Max sit-ups in 2:00
Max pull-ups in 2:00
Max flutterkicks in 2:00

Run

Run 1.5 mile

AIR FORCE PJ/CCT WORKOUT

WEEK 1

THURSDAY

Warm-Up and Stretch: 5:00

Swim Techniques

Tread water, no hands:
   5 times 1:00
Bobbing: 5:00
Floating: 5:00
Buddy breathing with
   snorkel: 5:00

Underwater Swimming
   (Note: Do not do this alone.)
   5 times 25 meters

FRIDAY

Warm-Up and Stretch: 5:00

Run

1.5-mile timed run

Swim

2 times 500-yard CSS timed
1000-meter swim with fins

SATURDAY

Warm-Up and Stretch: 5:00

PT

Max flutterkicks 1:00
Max push-ups in 2:00
Max sit-ups in 2:00
Max pull-ups

Pyramid to Failure

Pull-ups times 1
Push-ups times 3
Abs times 5

See page 114. Start at bottom,
go to max sets in all events,
and then back to the bottom.
If you fail in one event, pull-
ups for example, before the
others, just do negatives or
assisteds until you max on
two of the three events.

Run

1.5-mile timed run

WEEK 2

AIR FORCE PJ/CCT WORKOUT

MONDAY

Warm-Up and Stretch: 5:00

Full-Body / Push-Pull PT

Repeat 10 times:
Push-ups	40
Squats	40
Lunges	10/leg
Pull-ups	max or 10
Calve raises	40
Sit-ups	25

Abs / Lower Back PT

Repeat 3 times:
Flutterkicks	50
Crunches	50
Sit-ups	50
Supermans	1:00

Run

4-mile run

TUESDAY

Warm-Up and Stretch: 5:00

Run / Swim / Run

Run: 3 miles
Swim: 20:00 sprint (swim CSS at least 1000m)
Pool Drills: 20:00
Run: 1.5 miles

WEDNESDAY

Warm-Up and Stretch: 5:00

Swim / PT

Pull-ups: 100 reps in as few sets as possible

2000m Hypoxic Pyramid (see page 115): 100m x 2, 4, 6, 8, 10 strokes per breath

Pull-ups:	Max
Sit-ups:	50
Bent over rows:	20/arm

Pool work: 15:00 CSS

AIR FORCE PJ/CCT WORKOUT

WEEK 2

THURSDAY

Warm-Up and Stretch:	5:00

PT

Repeat 5 times:

Bench press:	20
Flutterkicks:	50
Sit-ups:	50
Push-ups:	50
Crunches:	50
Supermans:	20
Side bends:	20

Cardio

Bike or Run: 30:00

FRIDAY

Warm-Up and Stretch:	5:00

Run / Swim / Run

Run 4 miles or bike 30:00

2000m Hypoxic Pyramid: 200m times 2, 4, 6, 8, 10, 10, 8, 6, 4, 2 strokes per breath.

Pool drills: 15:00

Cardio

1.5-mile timed run or 15:00 biking

SATURDAY

Warm-Up and Stretch:	5:00

Run / Leg PT

Jog: 1 mile
Sprint: 1/4 mile
Squats: 40
Lunges: 20/leg
Jog: 1/4 mile in 2:00
Sprint: 1/4 mile
Squats: 40
Lunges: 20/leg
Jog: 1/4 mile in 2:00
Sprint: 1/8 mile
Squats: 40
Lunges: 20 /leg
Jog: 1/8 mile in 1:00
Sprint: 1/8 mile
Squats: 40
Lunges: 20/leg
Jog: 1/8 mile in 1:00

Swim PT

1000m Hypoxic Pyramid: 100m times 4 6, 8, 10, 12, 14, 12, 10, 8, 6 strokes per breath

Push-ups	20
Flutterkicks	25

200m CSS cool down

WEEK 3

AIR FORCE PJ/CCT WORKOUT

MONDAY

Warm-Up and Stretch: 5:00

Hypoxic swim / PT

Repeat 10 times:
Swim	100m
Push-ups	20
Flutterkicks	25

Each 100m swim should be 1000m Hypoxic Pyramid: 100m times 2, 4, 6, 8, 10, 10, 8, 6, 4, 2 strokes per breath

Stretch

Pull-ups: 100 any way you can: 10 times 10; 5 times 20—your choice

TUESDAY

Warm-Up and Stretch: 5:00

Swim

1000m Hypoxic Pyramid: 100m times 2, 4, 6, 8, 10, 10, 8, 6, 4, 2 strokes per breath

PT

Repeat 3 times:
Crunches:	100
Flutterkicks:	100
Leg levers:	100

WEDNESDAY

Warm-Up and Stretch: 5:00

Swim

Swim with fins: 500m
Swim w/o fins: 500m timed

Swim / PT

1000m Hypoxic Pyramid: 2, 4, 6, 8, 10, 10, 8, 6, 4, 2 strokes per breath

Push-ups:	20
Crunches:	30

Pool Drills: 15:00 CSS

Pull-Up PT

Regular grip:	2, 4, 6, 8, 10

100 abs of your choice
Reverse grip:	2, 4, 6, 8

100 abs of your choice
Wide grip:	2, 4, 6, 8

100 abs of your choice
Close grip:	2, 4, 6, 8

100 abs of your choice

AIR FORCE PJ/CCT WORKOUT

WEEK 3

THURSDAY

Warm-Up and Stretch: 5:00

Lower Body PT

Repeat 4 times:
Bike or glide*:	5:00
Squats:	20
Half squats:	20
Lunges:	10/leg

* Bike or use elliptical glider at high resistance levels, such as 10 to 15 out of 20 levels.

FRIDAY

Warm-Up and Stretch: 5:00

Bike, swim, or glide: 30:00

Repeat 2 times:
Pull-ups:	Max
Flutterkicks:	100
Push-ups:	Max
Sit-ups:	Max
Pull-ups:	
Wide grip:	10
...Regular grip:	10
...Reverse grip:	10
Crunches:	100

Pool Drills: 15:00

SATURDAY

Warm-Up and Stretch: 5:00

Run / Swim / PT / Bike

Run: 1.5-mile test
1000m Hypoxic Pyramid:
100m times 2, 4, 6, 8, 10, 10, 8, 6, 4, 2 strokes per breath

After each 100m:
Push-ups:	20
Crunches:	20

Pool Drills:	15:00
Run:	30:00

WEEK 4   AIR FORCE PJ/CCT WORKOUT

MONDAY

1.5-mile Warm-Up Jog/Stretch

Upperbody PT
Pull-ups:
Regular grip:	2, 4, 6, 8, 10
Reverse grip:	2, 4, 6, 8, 10
Wide grip:	2, 4, 6, 8
Close grip:	2, 4, 6, 8

Swim / PT
1000m Hypoxic Pyramid:
100m times 2, 4, 6, 8, 10, 10, 8, 6, 4, 2 strokes per breath

Push-ups:	20
Flutterkicks:	20

Pool drills:	20:00

TUESDAY

Warm-Up and Stretch:	5:00

Swim
500m CSS
500m with fins
3 x 100m sprints
4 x 50m sprints
Rest ::15 each 50m
200m cool down

Pool drills:	20:00

Run
3-mile track workout (see Thursday)

Stretch

WEDNESDAY

Warm-Up, Jog, Stretch:	5:00

Upperbody PT
Pull-ups:
Regular grip:	2, 4, 6, 8, 10
Reverse grip:	2, 4, 6, 8, 10
Close grip:	2, 4, 6, 8, 10
Wide grip:	2, 4, 6, 8, 10
Mountain climber:	2, 4, 6, 8, 10

Swim PT
Repeat 10 times:
Swim 100m CSS at
1:40 to 2:00

1000m Hypoxic Pyramid: 100m times 2, 4, 6, 8, 10, 10, 8, 6, 4, 2 strokes per breath

After each set do:
Push-ups:	20
Flutterkicks:	20

AIR FORCE PJ/CCT WORKOUT

WEEK 4

THURSDAY

Warm-Up and Stretch: 5:00

Swim

1000m Hypoxic Pyramid:
100m times 2, 4, 6, 8, 10, 10, 8, 6, 4, 2 strokes per breath

Run

3-mile track workout:

Jog:	1 mile
Sprint:	1/4 mile
Jog:	1/4 mile in 2:00
Sprint:	1/4 mile
Jog:	1/4 mile in 2:00
Sprint:	1/8 mile
Jog:	1/8 mile in 1:00
Sprint:	1/8 mile
Jog:	1/8 mile in 1:00
Sprint:	1/8 mile
Jog:	1/8 mile in 1:00
Sprint:	1/8 mile
Jog:	1/8 mile in 1:00

FRIDAY

Warm-Up and Stretch: 5:00

No Run Day

Back / Lower Body PT

Repeat 3 times:

Bike or run:	5:00
Pull-ups:	max
Squats:	50
Pull-ups:	max
Lunges:	20/leg
Pull-ups:	max
Calves:	50
Pull-ups:	max
Flutterkicks:	100

Swim

1000m swim:
  500m CSS swim
  500m choice of stroke

Pool drills: 20:00

SATURDAY

1.5-mile Warm-Up Jog, Stretch

Swim

500m sidestroke
1000-yard Hypoxic Pyramid: 2, 4, 6, 8, 10, 10, 8, 6, 4, 2 strokes per breath times 100 yds.
200m cool down

Upperbody PT

Max push-ups in 2:00
Max Situps in 2:00
Max push-ups in 1:30
Max sit-ups in 1:30
Max push-ups in 1:00
Max sit-ups in 1:00
Max push-ups in :30
Max sit-ups in :30
Max pushup in :15
Max sit-ups in :15

Ab PT

Sit-ups	100
Leg levers	50
Flutterkicks	50
Supermans	1:00

WEEK 5   AIR FORCE PJ/CCT WORKOUT

MONDAY

Warm-Up and Stretch: 5:00

Run / Leg PT

Jog:	1 mile
Sprint:	1/4 mile
Squats:	40
Lunges:	20/leg
Jog:	1/4 mile in 2:00
Sprint:	1/4 mile
Squats:	40
Lunges:	20/leg
Jog:	1/4 mile in 2:00
Sprint:	1/8 mile
Squats:	40
Lunges:	20/leg
Jog:	1/8 mile in 1:00
Sprint:	1/8 mile
Squats:	40
Lunges:	20/leg
Jog:	1/8 mile in 1:00

PT

Repeat 5 times:
   Max sit-ups in 2:00
   Max push-ups in 2:00

TUESDAY

Warm-Up and Stretch: 5:00

PT

Pull-ups: 100 in as few set as possible

Swim

Hypoxic: 200m times 10, 2, 4, 6, 8, 10, 10, 8, 6, 4, 2 stroke per breath

WEDNESDAY

Warm-Up and Stretch: 5:00

Rest Day

AIR FORCE PJ/CCT WORKOUT   WEEK 5

THURSDAY

Warm-Up and Stretch: 5:00

Swim

2000m Hypoxic Pyramid: 200m times 10, 2, 4, 6, 8, 10, 10, 8, 6, 4, 2 strokes per breath

Repeat 10 times:
  25yd CSS, easy
  25yd underwater. Do not do alone.

Pull-Up / Ab PT

Pull-ups:	max
Sit-ups or crunches:	100
Pull-ups:	max – 2
Sit-ups or crunches:	100
Pull-ups	max – 4
Sit-ups or crunches:	100
Pull-ups:	max – 6
Sit-ups or crunches:	100
Pull-ups:	max – 8
Sit-ups or crunches:	100
Pull-ups:	max – 10
Sit-ups or crunches:	100
Pull-ups:	max – 12
Sit-ups or crunches:	100

FRIDAY

Warm-Up and Stretch: 5:00

Run / Swim / Run

Run 3 miles or bike 30:00

Swim 2000m:
  1000m with fins
  1000m w/out fins

Run 1.5 miles timed
  or bike 15:00

SATURDAY

Warm-Up and Stretch: 5:00

PT

Pull-ups: 150 in as few sets as possible
Push-ups: 50 between each pull-up set

Rest with 100 abs of choice each set

WEEK 6

AIR FORCE PJ/CCT WORKOUT

MONDAY

Warm-Up and Stretch: 5:00

PJ/CCT Test

500yd timed CSS

Max flutterkicks in 2:00
Max push-ups in 2:00
Rest 2:00
Max sit-ups or crunches
   in 2:00
Rest 2:00
Max pull-ups

1.5-mile sprint

TUESDAY

Rest Day

WEDNESDAY

Warm-Up and Stretch: 5:00

Swim Test

500yd CSS
Rest / stretch: 5:00
500yd freestyle

PT

2:00 each:
   Max push-ups
   Max sit-ups
   Max pull-ups
   Max flutterkicks

Run

1.5-mile run

AIR FORCE PJ/CCT WORKOUT WEEK 6

THURSDAY

Warm-Up and Stretch: 5:00

Pool Technique
Treading water, no hands:
  1:00

5:00 of each:
  Bobbing
  Floating
  Buddy breathing w/ snorkel

Underwater Swims:
  Note: Do not do alone.
  25m x 5

FRIDAY

Warm-Up and Stretch: 5:00

Run
1.5 mile-timed run

Swim
500yd CSS timed x 2
1000m swim with fins

Pool drills: 20:00

SATURDAY

Warm-Up and Stretch: 5:00

Swim
500yd CSS
Pool drills: 20:00

Max flutterkicks in 1:00
Max push-ups in 2:00
Max sit-ups in 2:00
Max pull-ups

Pyramid to Failure
Pull-ups x 1
Push-ups x 3
Abs x 5

See page 114. Start at bottom, go to max sets in all events, and then back to the bottom. If you fail in one event, dips for example, before the others, just do negatives or assisteds until you max on two of the three events.

Run
1.5-mile timed

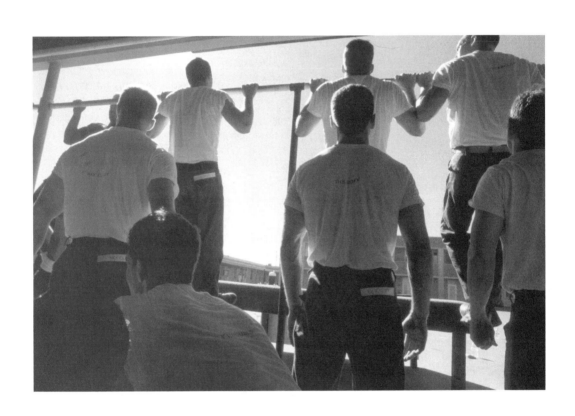

★ NAVY SEAL WORKOUT

WEEK 1   NAVY SEAL WORKOUT

MONDAY

Warm-Up and Stretch: 5:00

Upper Body PT
10 Supersets:
Pullups:	10 to 20
Abs of choice:	50
Dips:	20

Abs
2 Supersets:
Hanging knee-ups	25
Regular sit-ups	50
Flutterkicks:	50
Crunches:	50
Medicine ball sit-ups:	25

Optional: Do sit-ups / crunches with 25 lb dumbbell on your chest.

Swim 500m CSS

1000m Hypoxic Pyramid: 100m times 10, 2, 4, 6, 8, 10, 10, 8, 6, 4, 2 strokes per breath

2-mile sprint

TUESDAY

Warm-Up and Stretch: 5:00

Run / PT
Run:	15:00
Push-ups:	100
Abs of choice:	100
Run:	15:00
Push-ups:	75
Abs of choice:	200
Run:	15:00
Push-ups:	50
Abs of choice:	300

Mix some 8-Count Body Builders into the push-up section, too.

Push-ups, anyway you can: wide, regular, knee. Like PFT, if possible.

1.5-mile run

WEDNESDAY

Warm-Up and Stretch: 5:00

Lower Body PT
Repeat 3 to 4 times:
Run	5:00
Squats:	1:00
Lunges:	1:00
Calves:	1:00

PT Pyramid

Pull-ups times 1
Push-ups times 2

PT Supersets
Repeat 10 times:
Pull-ups:	5 to 10
Push-ups:	20
Sit-ups:	20

Abs
2 Supersets:
Hanging knee-ups	25
Regular sit-ups	50
Flutterkicks:	50
Crunches:	50
Medicine ball sit-ups:	25

Optional: Do sit-ups or crunches with a 25lb dumbbell on your chest.

NAVY SEAL WORKOUT

WEEK 1

THURSDAY

Warm-Up and Stretch: 5:00

PT Day Off
Run

Run 30:00
1-mile repeats for 30:00 (try
for 4 miles at least)

Swim

1000m Hypoxic Pyramid: 100m
times 2, 4, 6, 8, 10, 10, 8, 6, 4, 2
strokes per breath

500yd CSS timed

Cooldown:
  100 breaststroke
  200yds just kicking
  200yds just arms

FRIDAY

Warm-Up and Stretch: 5:00

PT
Repeat 20 times:
  Jumping jacks: 20
  Push-ups: 20

Stretch

Shoulder press: 20
Woodchoppers: 20

Abs
2 Supersets:
  Hanging knee-ups   25
Regular sit-ups   50
  Flutterkicks: 50
  Crunches: 50
  Medicine ball sit-ups: 25

Optional: Do sit-ups / crunches with 25lb dumbbell on your
chest.

2000m Hypoxic Pyramid: 200m
times 2, 4, 6, 8, 10, 10, 8, 6, 4, 2
strokes per breath.

SATURDAY

Warm-Up and Stretch: 5:00

Run/PT
Run:	15:00
Squats:	100
Abs of choice:	100
Run:	15:00
Lunges:	75
Abs of choice:	75
Run:	15:00
Half squats:	50
Abs of choice:	50

Long-distance swim:2 miles,
CSS with fins

WEEK 2 NAVY SEAL WORKOUT

MONDAY

Warm-Up and Stretch:	5:00

2-Mile Run

Repeat 4 times:
  1/4-mile repeats

Repeat 8 times:
  1/8-mile repeats

Push-ups:	Max in 2:00
Rest:	2:00
Sit-ups:	Max in 2:00
Rest:	2:00
Push-ups:	Max in 1:00
Sit-ups:	Max in 1:00
Rest:	2:00
Push-ups:	Max in ::30
Sit-ups:	Max in ::30

More BUDS Abs

Flutterkicks:	100
Leg levers:	100
Sit-ups (with boots on):	100

TUESDAY

Warm-Up, Run, Stretch:	5:00

PT

Repeat 10 times:
Jumping jacks:	10
Squats:	20
Pull-ups:	10

(Mix some overhead squats and weighted squats in the sets.)

Repeat 6 times:
  Run: 1/2 mile repeats at sub 3:00 pace

Repeat 5 times:
Pull-ups (grip of your choice):	max
Squats:	30
Lunges: (your choice):	30

Abs

Repeat 2 times:
Sit-ups:	100
Flutterkicks:	100
Leg levers:	100

1000m Hypoxic Pyramid:
  100m times 4, 6, 8, 10, 12 strokes per breath (CSS)

1000m Hypoxic Pyramid:
  100m times 4, 6, 8, 10, 12 strokes per breath (Freestyle)

WEDNESDAY

Warm-Up and Stretch:	5:00

Run / Swim / PT

3-mile timed run:
  3 1-mile repeats

Swim with fins:	1000m

Repeat 10 times:
Push-ups:	20
Sit-ups:	40
Triceps push-ups:	20
Reverse crunches:	40

Swim 100m timed

Hypoxic Swim PT

1000m Hypoxic Swim:
  100m times 2, 4, 6, 8, 10, 12, 14, 12, 10, 8, 6, 4, 2 strokes per breath (CSS, timed)

1000m Hypoxic Swim:
  100m times 2, 4, 6, 8, 10, 12, 14, 12, 10, 8, 6, 4, 2 strokes per breath

Push-ups:	20
Abs of choice:	20

NAVY SEAL WORKOUT

WEEK 2

THURSDAY

Warm-Up and Stretch: 5:00

Back / Legs

Repeat 3 times:
Squats:	30
Pull-ups:	
Regular:	10
Reverse:	10

Run 1 mile, 6:00 pace
Squats:	40

Run 1 mile, 6:00 pace
Lunges:	40/leg

run 1 mile 6:00 pace
Squats:	40

Run 1 mile, 6:00 pace
Lunges:	40/leg

Do your best to keep to a 6:00 pace

FRIDAY

Warm-Up and Stretch: 5:00

Hypoxic Swim PT

1000m Hypoxic Swim:
100m times 2, 4, 6, 8, 10, 12, 14, 12, 10, 8, 6, 4, 2 strokes per breath (CSS, timed)

1000m Hypoxic Swim:
100m times 2, 4, 6, 8, 10, 12, 14, 12, 10, 8, 6, 4, 2 strokes per breath

Push-ups:	20
Abs of choice:	20

SATURDAY

Warm-Up and Stretch: 5:00

Run / Swim / PT
Repeat 2 times:
  1/2-mile sprint
  1/4-mile jog

Repeat 4 times:
  1/4-mile sprint
  1/8-mile jog

Repeat 8 times:
  1/8-mile sprint
  1/8-mile jog

SUNDAY

PT Pyramid

Pull-ups times 1
Push-ups times 2
Sit-ups times 5

See page 114. Start at bottom, go to 10 sets in all events, and then back to the bottom.

Repeat 10 times:
Jumping jacks:	10
Push-ups:	10

WEEK 3

NAVY SEAL WORKOUT

MONDAY

Warm-Up and Stretch: 5:00

Rest Day

This week, try to make a 6:00 per mile pace on all track workouts:

    1/4 mile: ::90
    1/2 mile: 3:00

TUESDAY

Warm-Up and Stretch: 5:00

Pull-Ups

Regular grip: 2, 4, 6, 8, 10, 8, 6, 4, 2
Reverse grip: 2, 4, 6, 8, 10, 8, 6, 4, 2
Close grip: 2, 4, 6, 8, 10, 8, 6, 4, 2
Wide grip: 2, 4, 6, 8, 10, 8, 6, 4, 2

Abs of choice: 20 between each set of pull-ups
    200 pull-ups
    720 abs

Track Workout

1/2-mile repeats times 6 (Walk 1/4 mile between repeats.)

Swim

1500m Hypoxic Pyramid:
    100m x 2, 4, 6, 8, 10, 12, 14, 16,14, 12, 10, 8, 6, 4, 2 strokes per breath. If nec essary, rest at each wall on higher hypoxics.

WEDNESDAY

Warm-Up and Stretch: 5:00

No Run Day

Repeat 4 times:
    Swim 500m CSS timed

Between each set of 500m:
    Max push-ups in 2:00
    Max sit-ups in 2:00

NAVY SEAL WORKOUT   WEEK 3

THURSDAY

Warm-Up and Stretch: 5:00

Pull-Ups
Regular grip:	2, 4, 6, 8, 10, 12
Reverse grip:	2, 4, 6, 8, 10, 12
Close grip:	2, 4, 6, 8, 10, 12
Wide grip:	2, 4, 6, 8, 10, 12

20 abs of choice between each set of pull-ups

Track Workout

1/4-mile repeats times 12 (Walk 1/8 mile between repeats)

FRIDAY

Warm-Up and Stretch: 5:00

Track Workout

1/8-mile repeats times 20 (Walk 100yds between repeats.)

PT Day Off

Easy swim: 1-mile CSS with fins

SATURDAY

Warm-Up and Stretch: 5:00

SEAL PFT

500m swim	
Rest:	10:00
Push-ups:	Max
Rest:	2:00
Sit-ups:	Max
Rest:	2:00
Pull-ups:	Max
Rest:	10:00

1.5-mile run

WEEK 4

NAVY SEAL WORKOUT

MONDAY

3-mile Warm-Up Jog/ Stretch

Pull-Ups
Regular grip: 2, 4, 6, 8, 10, 12
Reverse grip: 2, 4, 6, 8, 10, 12
Close grip: 2, 4, 6, 8, 10, 12
Wide grip: 2, 4, 6, 8, 10, 12

Swim / PT

Repeat 10 times:
  100m freestyle
  20 push-ups
  20 abs of choice

TUESDAY

Warm-Up and Stretch: 5:00

Swim

500m CSS
500m CSS with fins
3 times 100m sprints
4 times 50m sprints
(rest ::15 each 50m)

200m cool-down

3-mile Track Workout:

Jog:	1 mile
Sprint:	1/4 mile
Jog:	1/4 mile in 2:00
Sprint:	1/4 mile
Jog:	1/4 mile in 2:00
Sprint:	1/8 mile
Jog:	1/8 mile in 1:00
Sprint:	1/8 mile
Jog:	1/8 mile in 1:00
Sprint:	1/8 mile
Jog:	1/8 mile in 1:00
Sprint:	1/8 mile
Jog:	1/8 mile in 1:00

WEDNESDAY

Warm-Up and Stretch: 5:00

Upperbody PT
Pull-Ups
Regular grip: 2, 4, 6, 8, 10, 12
Reverse grip: 2, 4, 6, 8, 10, 12
Close grip: 2, 4, 6, 8, 10, 12
Wide grip: 2, 4, 6, 8, 10, 12
Towel grip: 2, 4, 6, 8, 10, 12

Swim PT

1000m Hypoxic Pyramid: 100m
times 2, 4, 6, 8, 10, 10, 8, 6, 4, 2
strokes per breath

Push-ups:	20
Abs of choice:	20

NAVY SEAL WORKOUT

WEEK 4

THURSDAY

Warm-Up and Stretch: 5:00

Swim

2000m Hypoxic Pyramid:
200m x 2, 4, 6, 8, 10, 10, 8, 6, 4,
2 strokes per breath

Run

3-mile Track Workout:

Jog:	1 mile
Sprint:	1/4 mile
Jog:	1/4 mile in 2:00
Sprint:	1/4 mile
Jog:	1/4 mile in 2:00
Sprint:	1/8 mile
Jog:	1/8 mile in 1:00
Sprint:	1/8 mile
Jog:	1/8 mile in 1:00
Sprint:	1/8 mile
Jog:	1/8 mile in 1:00
Sprint:	1/8 mile
Jog:	1/8 mile in 1:00

FRIDAY

Warm-Up and Stretch: 5:00

Back / Lowerbody PT

Repeat 3 times

Run or bike:	5:00
Max pull-ups	
Squats:	50
Max pull-ups	
Lunge:	20/leg
Max pull-ups	
Calves:	50
Max pull-ups	
Flutterkicks:	100

(12 sets of max pull-ups = total)

Swim

1000m swim
500m swim
500m swim with fins

SATURDAY

3-mile Warm-Up Jog/ Stretch

Swim

500m CSS
3 times 100m sprints
(rest ::30 after each 100)
4 times 50m sprints
(rest ::15 after each 50m)
200m cool-down

Upperbody PT

Push-ups:	Max in 2:00
Sit-ups:	Max in 2:00
Push-ups:	Max in 1:30
Sit-ups:	Max in 1:30
Push-ups:	Max in 1:00
Sit-ups:	Max in 1:00
Push-ups:	Max in ::30
Sit-ups:	Max in ::30
Push-ups:	Max in ::15
Sit-ups:	Max in ::15

WEEK 5 NAVY SEAL WORKOUT

MONDAY

Warm-Up and Stretch: 5:00

PT / Run

Repeat 10 times:
- Jumping jacks: 10
- Push-ups: 10

Run:	1.5 miles
Push-ups:	50
Sit-ups:	100
Run:	1.5 miles
Push-ups:	50
Sit-ups:	100
Sprint:	1.5 miles
Push-ups:	50
Sit-ups:	100

500m Hypoxic Pyramid:
100 times 4, 6, 8, 10, 12 strokes per breath (CSS)

500m Hypoxic Pyramid:
100 times 4, 6, 8, 10, 12 strokes per breath (Freestyle)

TUESDAY

Warm-Up and Stretch: 5:00

Pull Ups / Downs

Repeat 6 times:
- Pull-ups: Max
- Bent-over rows: 10

Run / PT

Repeat 5 times:
- Sprint: 5:00
- Squats: 40
- Lunges: 20 / leg

Stretch

WEDNESDAY

Warm-Up and Stretch: 5:00

Supersets

Repeat 20 times:
- Sit-ups: 10
- Push-ups: 10
- Rev crunches: 10
- Triceps push-ups: 10
- Leg levers: 10
- Wide push-ups: 10

(Try to do each cycle of each exercises in 2:00)

Totals in 40:00:
600 abs
600 push-ups

Jog 30:00

500m Hypoxic Pyramid:
100 times 4, 6, 8, 10, 12 strokes per breath (CSS)

500m Hypoxic Pyramid:
100 times 4, 6, 8, 10, 12 strokes per breath (Freestyle)

NAVY SEAL WORKOUT

WEEK 5

THURSDAY

Warm-Up and Stretch: 5:00

Rest Day

FRIDAY

Warm-Up and Stretch: 5:00

Testing Day

Repeat 2 times:
Push-ups:	Max in 2:00
Sit-ups:	Max in 2:00
Pull-ups:	Max

Run:	1.5 miles
Swim:	500yd

500m Hypoxic Pyramid:
100 times 4, 6, 8, 10, 12
strokes per breath (CSS)

500m Hypoxic Pyramid:
100 times 4, 6, 8, 10, 12
strokes per breath
(Freestyle)

Run: 1.5 miles

SATURDAY

Warm-Up and Stretch: 5:00

Recovery Day

Rest and stretch

SUNDAY

Rest or swim 500yd timed CSS

WEEK 6

NAVY SEAL WORKOUT

MONDAY

Warm-Up and Stretch: 5:00

Navy SEAL PFT

500m swim
Push-ups: Max in 2:00
Sit-ups: Max in 2:00
Pull-ups   Max
Run: 1.5 mile

Pull-Up Pyramid

Regular grip times 1
Reverse grip times 1

50 abs of choice between
each set of abs

Totals:
   Abs = 600
   Pull-ups = 100-plus

TUESDAY

Warm-Up and Stretch: 5:00

Run / Swim / Run

Run: 3 miles
Swim: 1 mile
Run: 3 miles

Swim
   1000m with fins
   1000m w/o fins (CSS)

WEDNESDAY

Warm-Up and Stretch: 5:00

Pull-ups

Regular grip: 2, 4, 6, 8, 10,
   8, 6, 4, 2
Reverse grip: 2, 4, 6, 8, 10,
   8, 6, 4, 2
Close grip: 2, 4, 6, 8, 10,
   8, 6, 4, 2
Wide grip: 2, 4, 6, 8, 10,
   8, 6, 4, 2
Towel pull-ups: 2, 4, 6, 8, 10,
   8, 6, 4, 2

Total:
   250 pull-ups

Push-ups: Max in 2:00
Sit-ups: Max in 2:00

Repeat sets, decreasing number of sit-ups and push-ups by
10 until you are at 0 push-ups
and 0 sit-ups.

AL WORKOUT

WEEK 6

DAY

retch: 5:00

00

Max in 1:00
Max in 1:00
Max in 1:00

Swim

Warm-up: 200m
CSS: 500m

500m Hypoxic Pyramid:
  50m times 2, 4, 6, 8, 10, 12,
  14, 16, 18, 20 strokes per
  length. Breathe at walls.

500m with fins
200m cool down

FRIDAY

Warm-Up and Stretch: 5:00

Bike or Run
30:00

Rest and Stretch

SATURDAY

Warm-Up and Stretch: 5:00

LEG PT
Repeat 4 times:
  Run: 1/2 mile in 3:00
  Squats: Max in 1:00
  Lunges: Max in 1:00
  Heel raises: Max in 1:00

Swim

Warm-up: 200m
CSS: 500m

500m Hypoxic Pyramid:
  50m times 2, 4, 6, 8, 10, 12,
  14, 16, 18, 20 strokes per
  length. Breathe at walls.

500m with fins
2000m swim:
  1000m with fins
  1000m w/o fins (CSS)
200m cool down

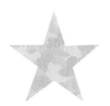

PART III:
SPECIAL OPS
NUTRITION

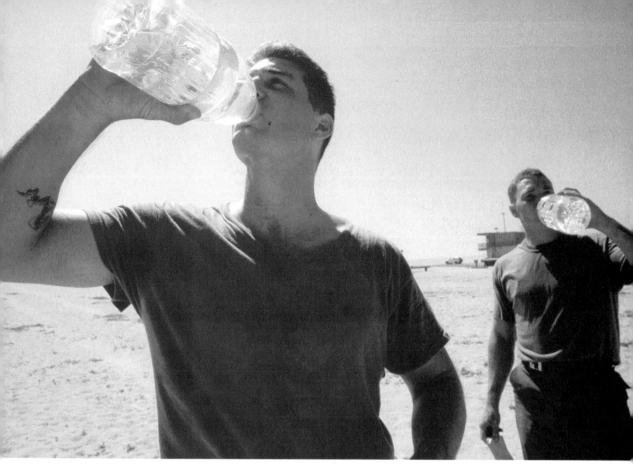

SPECIAL OPS NUTRITION

YOU CAN'T ACHIEVE PEAK FITNESS WITHOUT PAYING ATTENTION to what you eat. Strong dietary habits are critical both before entering training and during the training itself. Optimum performance is achieved by proper nutrient intake and is essential to receiving maximum performance output during exercise. Nutrition also promotes vital muscle and tissue growth and repair. The ideal diet provides all the nutrients that the body needs and supplies energy for exercise.

Balancing energy intake and expenditure can be very difficult when activity levels are very high (as in SOF training) and when activity levels are very low, such as during isolation. Typically, body weight remains constant when energy intake equals expenditure.

If Caloric Intake =	And Caloric Output =	The Result Is
3000	3000	No Change in Weight
4000	2000	Weight Gain
2000	3000	Weight Loss

You can upset this "energy balance equation" by increasing or decreasing the number of calories you consume, increasing or decreasing your energy expenditure, or both. One pound of body fat is equal to 3,500 calories. So to lose 1 pound in 1 week, you'd have to, over the course of the week, consume 3,500 fewer calories, increase your activity level, or a combination of the two. To gain 1 pound in the same time, you'd need to consume 3,500 calories more than you expend, decrease your physical activity, or a combination of both.

COMPONENTS OF ENERGY EXPENDITURE

The three major contributors to energy expenditure are:

* ★ Resting energy expenditure (REE)
* ★ Physical activity
* ★ Energy used to digest foods

The first two contributors are most pertinent to our discussion. Resting energy expenditure (REE) is the amount of energy required to maintain life—your breathing, heartbeat, body temperature regulation, and other vital processes (but not physical exertion). You can estimate your REE with the following formula.

Determining Resting Energy Expenditure (REE) of Men from Body Weight (in Pounds)

AGE (YEARS)	EQUATION TO DERIVE REE (CAL/DAY)
18 to 30	$6.95 \times \text{Weight} + 679$
30 to 60	$5.27 \times \text{Weight} + 879$

To calculate your *total* daily caloric expenditure you need to account for your physical activity in addition to your REE. The amount of energy expended during special forces training varies from day to day. Some days are very strenuous and involve running, swimming, calisthenics, cold water exposure, sleep deprivation, and carrying heavy loads. Some days are spent in the classroom sitting a good portion of the time. Thus, determining your actual energy expenditure during activity is more difficult. But there are ways to estimate. One is to multiply your REE by an "activity factor."

Estimating Total Daily Energy Needs of Men at Various Levels of Activity

LEVEL OF GENERAL ACTIVITY	ACTIVITY FACTOR
Very Light. Seated and standing activities, driving, playing cards	1.3
Light. Walking, carpentry, sailing, ping-pong, pool, or golf	1.6
Moderate. Carrying a load, jogging, light swimming, biking, calisthenics, scuba diving	1.7
Heavy. Walking with a load uphill, rowing, digging, climbing, soccer, basketball, running, obstacle course	2.1
Exceptional. Running/swimming races, biking uphill, carrying very heavy loads, hard rowing	2.4

Here's an example using a 21-year-old male who weighs 175 pounds and whose activity level is moderate:

REE = 6.95 x 175[1] + 679 = 1,895 calories per day
Total Energy Needs = 1895 x 1.7[2] = **3,222 calories per day**

[1] 175 = weight in pounds
[2] 1.7 = "Moderate" Activity Factor

BODY MASS INDEX

The Body Mass Index (BMI) is a measure commonly used to assess body composition and then classify individuals as underweight, overweight, or overfat. The BMI is a ratio: weight/height^2, with weight measured in kilograms and height in meters.

The reference ranges developed for the United States population as a whole do not always apply to special populations such as the men in special operations forces. For that reason, a BMI reference range based on a survey of 800 SEALs was developed. For all SEALs combined, for example, the average BMI was 25 and the average body fat was 13 percent. What is important to remember is that the index is a screening tool. You can use the BMI to assess and keep track of changes in your body composition. If your BMI is high, have your body fat checked. If it's more than 20 percent, you need to take some action to lower your weight. Reference BMI values for you are provided below:

Reference BMI Values

Lean	<20
Typical	20 to 29
Overfat	29 to 32

EATING FOR OPTIMUM HEALTH

Once you know where you stand in terms of your BMI, caloric intake, and caloric expenditures, it's important to carefully consider your diet. The following section is dedicated to explaining the way to build a healthful diet. The information comes from the Dietary Guidelines for Americans released in 2000 by the U.S. Department of Agriculture and the U.S. Department of Health and Human Services. Top dietitians and scientists have studied the practicality and reliability of the data. It is tested, supported, and credentialed.

In this section you'll learn about basic nutrition: Your daily nutrient and caloric needs; vitamins, minerals, and more. From there you'll discover the Food Pyramid.

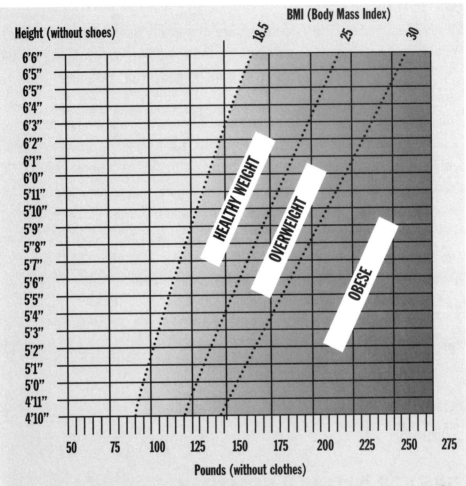

Height (without shoes) — BMI (Body Mass Index) — **Pounds (without clothes)**

HEALTHY WEIGHT   OVERWEIGHT   OBESE

BMI measures weight in relation to height. The BMI ranges shown above are for adults. They are not exact ranges of healthy and unhealthy weights. However, they show that health risk increases at higher levels of overweight and obesity. Even within the healthy BMI range, weight gains can carry health risks for adults.

Directions: Find your weight on the bottom of the graph. Go straight up from that point until you come to the line that matches your height. Then look to find your weight group.

Healthy Weight: BMI from 18.5 up to 25 refers to a healthy weight.
Overweight: BMI from 25 up to 30 refers to overweight.
Obese: BMI 30 or higher refers to obesity. Obese persons are also overweight.

It's a simple yet profound way to understand where your calories should come from. Finally, you'll learn how to read a nutrition label and be able to make intelligent, healthy decisions at the supermarket or even at a fast food restaurant.

THE CHALLENGE OF CHOICE

Good nutrition boils down to two elements: choice and portion size. Choice involves the types of foods you eat and how they're prepared. Are you more apt to eat a baked sweet potato or a plate of fries? An apple or apple pie? Even the simplest choices, such as the decision to forego slabs of butter on your pancakes, can save you hundreds of calories that you probably won't even miss in terms of flavor.

As important as *what* you eat is *how much* of each food you eat. There are no good or bad foods (with the exception of trans-fatty acids, which is covered later). Portion control is the key. In the last few years portion sizes of virtually all foods—from mega-muffins and "big grab" chips, to cookies, to restaurant entrees—have ballooned. Often, what is sold in single packages really represents two or three servings. In this section you'll also find out how to determine sensible portion sizes based on the Food Guide Pyramid model.

NUTRITION BASICS

Fad diets come and go, but basic science-backed nutrition advice has remained remarkably consistent. In fact, many reported studies have proven that the best way to lose fat, keep it off, and enjoy a healthful diet is to follow a plan that is rooted not in a new trend, but in the Department of Agriculture's Food Guide Pyramid. While most of us are excited by new trends and fads, the truth is that they don't work in the long term. What does work is a balanced eating and exercising plan that is based on reasonable and attainable goals.

The key to the Food Guide Pyramid is that it provides a wide range of choices so you can eat a variety of tasty foods. Eating a variety of foods ensures that you get all the important nutrients, vitamins, and minerals that your body requires for optimal health. It also means that you won't be bored to death because you can select different foods every day.

★ STEW SMITH'S WEIGHT GAIN TIPS ★

It is up to you whether you gain or lose weight. To gain a pound a week you need to create a surplus of 3,500 calories more than you expend. If you think about this in terms of days and you only need to eat an additional 500 calories a day to gain a pound a week. Depending on your overall caloric intake, you can use this program to either lose or gain weight. The goal is to find something that you enjoy doing—whether it's running, walking, swimming, calisthenics, or weight training—and do it. If you don't enjoy your workout, chances are you won't continue the program.

HOW TO GAIN WEIGHT!

Gaining weight isn't easy to do; you probably already know this. People who cannot gain weight usually have a fast metabolism, which makes gaining hard. The key to weight gain is to do everything BIG.

You have to eat big and lift big, to get big.

This is your new motto! A lot of people think weightlifting is the key to gaining weight. It is an extremely important part; *however,* just as important is your diet. In fact, you can still do your calisthenics (PT) workouts and still gain weight, as long as you eat BIG.

So, to put it as simply as possible, here are 6 simple steps to follow if you want to bulk up:

1. Count how many calories you eat in a normal day. Don't change anything, just eat like you normally would and count how many calories you consumed. This is an extremely important step, so try to be as exact as possible. Also, weigh yourself.

2. Starting the day after you counted calories, eat 500 calories *more* than you normally do. For example, if you counted 2,000 calories on

one day, your would need to eat 2,500 calories a day. Instead of eating 3 big meals a day or eating all day all the time, spread those calories out over 5 or 6 smaller meals. Eat one meal every 2 and a half to 3 hours. To get big, you have to eat big! Remember that.

3. Weightlifting and rucking utilize the bigger muscles groups of the body including legs, butt, and lower back. This will spur growth to those muscles as well—this is where you should see your greatest increase in weight.

4. At the end of the week, weigh yourself. You'll notice you are gaining just after one week! Now, don't expect to see a 10-pound increase. Gaining anymore than 1 or 2 pounds a week is unhealthy and means you are putting on way too much fat. So look for 1or 2 pound gains at the end of the week. Doesn't sound like much? You can be gaining 5-8 pounds a month! A 10-pound weight gain will help as long as it does not impact your running, pull-ups, and other PT tests. So you have to keep working out harder in order to carry this extra weight.

5. Here's an important one. Eventually, you will stop seeing weight gain. At this point, you will have to eat even more. So, when you stop gaining for at least 2 weeks, it's time to start eating an extra 250 calories a day. Every time you see you haven't gained weight for at least 2 weeks, add an extra 250 calories, but only until you reach your goal.

6. Now, even more important: Keep working out. Do not just eat to get big. Lift to get big!

MORE WEIGHT-GAINING TIPS

Stay away from fat! Even though weight gain is your goal, you don't want to be gaining fat. Get rid of the chips and high-fat junk food. No more fast food, nothing fried. Stick to high-protein, low-fat foods like tuna fish (and other seafood), chicken breast, turkey, ham, lean meats, fruits, and vegetables.

Below is a list of foods you want to eat to gain weight:

Bagels	**Cream based soup**	Peanut butter and jelly
Beans, Peas	**Croissant**	**Peanuts**
Burgers	Fish	**Porterhouse steak**
Carrots	Ham Steak	Potatoes
Cheese	**Ice Cream**	**Prime rib steak**
Chicken	**Mayonnaise**	Raisin Bran cereal
Club sandwiches	**Milkshakes**	**Salad dressing**
Crackers	Oatmeal	

Eat the foods in **bold** in moderation, especially if you are trying to lose weight, because they are higher in fat. If you're trying to boost your caloric intake to 2,500 to 3,000 calories per day to gain weight. If you want to lose weight you have to drop your calories to 1,500 to 1,800 calories a day in addition to exercise.

Drink water! Drink around a gallon a day, more if you can. Yes, that's a lot of water, but it's water that will give you the energy you need to gain weight!

Fatigue and hunger are challenging issues you will have to handle. But making sound decisions and remaining calm while tired and hungry adds to the true test of leadership.

DAILY NUTRIENT NEEDS

For a healthy, balanced diet, you need to consume healthful portions of protein, carbohydrates, and fats. Here's the breakdown.

PROTEIN

Protein is made up of chemicals called amino acids. Some types of amino acids called *nonessential amino acids*—are produced by the body. Nine *essential amino acids* must come from food you consume. Protein allows the body to build, maintain, and replace body tissue. Muscles, organs, and some hormones are made up primarily of protein. Protein also makes hemoglobin—the part of red blood cells that carries oxygen—and antibodies, the cells that fight off infection and disease.

Good sources of protein include meat, chicken, fish, eggs, cheese, beans, and nuts.

The recommended intake of protein is 50 to 70 grams per day (which should equal 12 to 20 percent of your daily caloric intake).

CARBOHYDRATES

There are two types of carbohydrates: simple and complex. Simple carbohydrates are sugars. They're quickly and easily broken down and digested by the body. Complex carbohydrates, also known as starches, take longer to be digested than simple carbohydrates.

Carbohydrates are the preferred energy source for physical activity. It takes at least 20 hours after demanding exercise to restore muscle energy, provided 600 grams of carbohydrates are consumed each day. During successive days of exhausting training like that of SOF, your energy stores become depleted. A high-carbohydrate diet can help you maintain energy.

Good sources of simple carbohydrates include fruits, such as apples, bananas, grapes, raisins, oranges, and pears. Good sources of complex carbohydrates include bread, cereals, pasta, rice, oatmeal, pretzels, corn, potatoes, sweet potatoes, tomatoes, carrots, cucumbers, lettuce, and peppers.

Normally, the recommended intake of carbohydrates is 350 to 400 grams per day or 55 to 65 percent of your daily intake. During training, however, 600 grams per day or up to 70 percent of your daily caloric intake should be from carbohydrates. Most of that should be from foods high in complex carbohydrates (see above).

FAT

You'll notice that the Food Guide Pyramid allows you to consume 25 to 30 percent of your daily calories from fat. For too long Americans have bought into the myth that fat is evil and that as long as we severely restrict fat intake, we would also control weight. This was based largely on the fact that high-fat foods contain more calories per gram than do other foods. (A single gram of fat has 9 calories; a single gram of carbohydrates and protein has 4 calories.) However, substituting non-fat or low-fat products for fats has not led to success in fat loss. Why? Here are the facts about fat.

FACT: Fat-free does not equal calorie-free. Many non-fat or low-fat foods have very high levels of sugar, which often significantly increases the calorie content of foods. In addition, people tend to eat larger portions of fat-free foods, thereby increasing the amount of calories consumed.

FACT: Fat satiates. In general, you need to eat less of a food with fat than you do of a non-fat food to feel full. For this reason, many people tend to overeat non-fat or low-fat foods.

FACT: You *need* some fat. This one is hard for people to accept, but it is true. Fat is a major nutrient that is vital for proper growth and development and maintenance of good health. Certain vitamins (A, E, and K) are soluble only in fat.

However, not all fats are healthful. In general, you should steer clear of saturated fats, which are artery cloggers. You'll find them in butter, meats, and palm and coconut oils. You should also avoid trans-fatty acids (fats that are formed when foods are hydrogenated and which are found in deep fried commercial foods and many packaged foods, especially baked goods). These fats act like saturated fats but are even worse: In addition to raising levels of so-called "bad" cholesterol (known as LDL) in our bodies (as saturated fats do), they lower the levels of the "good" cholesterol (HDL) necessary to keep our arteries clear.

Monosaturated and polyunsaturated fats are the "good" fats. They're found in foods including olive oil and canola oil and are absolutely necessary for many functions of life. Our bodies also require essential fatty acids (EFAs), such as linoleic and alpha linoleic acid, for normal cell growth and development. The only way to get these fatty acids is through your diet. EFAs are found primarily in fatty fish, such as salmon and mackerel, and in certain nuts, oils, and dark green vegetables. There is significant evidence that a diet rich in essential fatty acids can protect against heart disease. Recently, the American Heart Association, in recognition of the important heart protective role that these fatty acids play, revised their dietary guidelines to include suggesting that we eat two servings of fatty fish each week.

Recommended daily intake of fat is 30 to 65 grams per day (approximately 25 to 30 percent of your caloric intake.).

THE FOOD GUIDE PYRAMID

The Food Guide Pyramid provides a visual depiction of the types and quantities of foods you should eat every day. It is broken into six food groups: grains, vegetables, fruits, dairy, proteins, and fats and sweets. Most of your diet should come from the foods at the base of the Pyramid (the grains group); the least amount should come from those at the top (fats, oils and sweets). You'll notice that you can have six to 11 servings of grains each day, which are rich in carbohydrates.

WHAT COUNTS AS A SERVING?

The Food Guide Pyramid tells us to eat a particular number of servings per day of each kind of food: 3 servings of meat, 3 servings of milk, and so forth. But what exactly is one serving?

MILK, YOGURT, AND CHEESE

Eat 2 to 3 servings every day
1 serving equals 1 1/2 ounces of natural cheese OR 2 ounces of process cheese OR 8 ounces of yogurt OR 8 ounces of milk.

FOOD GUIDE PYRAMID

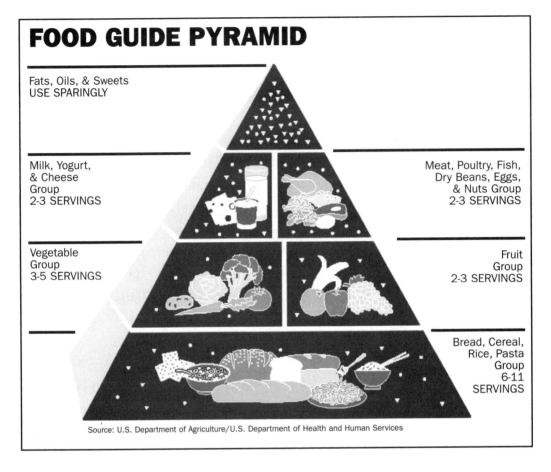

Fats, Oils, & Sweets
USE SPARINGLY

Milk, Yogurt,
& Cheese
Group
2-3 SERVINGS

Meat, Poultry, Fish,
Dry Beans, Eggs,
& Nuts Group
2-3 SERVINGS

Vegetable
Group
3-5 SERVINGS

Fruit
Group
2-3 SERVINGS

Bread, Cereal,
Rice, Pasta
Group
6-11
SERVINGS

Source: U.S. Department of Agriculture/U.S. Department of Health and Human Services

MEAT, POULTRY, FISH

Eat 2 to 3 servings every day

1 serving equals 2 to 3 ounces of cooked lean meat, poultry, or fish. 1/2 cup of cooked dry beans OR 1 egg OR 2 tablespoons peanut butter count as *1 ounce* of lean meat.

VEGETABLES

Eat 3 to 5 servings every day

1 serving equals 1 cup of raw leafy vegetables OR 1/2 cup of other vegetables, cooked or chopped raw OR 3/4 cup of vegetable juice.

FRUIT

Eat 2 to 4 servings every day

1 serving equals 1 medium apple, banana, or orange OR 1/2 cup of chopped, cooked, or canned fruit OR 3/4 cup of fruit juice.

CEREAL, RICE, AND PASTA

Eat 6 to 11 servings every day

1 serving equals 1 slice of bread OR 1 ounce of ready-to-eat cereal OR 1/2 cup of cooked cereal, rice, or pasta.

THE IMPORTANCE OF FRUITS AND VEGETABLES

In addition to choosing healthy grains, try to eat at least five servings of fruits and vegetables every day. This is essential. Many scientific studies have shown that people whose diets are plentiful in fruits and vegetables have reduced risk for many diseases, including a variety of cancers. Fruits and vegetables are great sources of essential vitamins, minerals, and fiber. Unfortunately, most of us do not eat the five recommended servings daily; and if we do, we eat the less healthy vegetables, such as iceberg lettuce, rather than the nutrient-dense dark greens. Dark green leafy vegetables, deeply colored fruits, and beans and peas are very rich in vitamins and minerals. A good rule of thumb is to make your plate as colorful as possible with a variety of vegetables to be sure you are getting all the nutrients you need.

How can you make sure you eat enough from this food group? Choose chopped vegetables as a snack when you feel hungry; or grab an apple instead of a candy bar. Drink juice instead of soda. Prepare salads with tomatoes, cucumbers, peppers, and other vegetables. Soon you'll see how easy it really is to eat those five servings.

WATER

Water, which comprises about 75 percent of our total body weight, serves many functions. It helps regulate our body temperature. When we sweat, we rid ourselves of excess heat. Water transports needed nutrients to our cells and removes toxic substances and wastes. It cushions our body tissues and lubricates our joints. Water provides moisture for our respiratory system and is essential for our digestion. Since water is a major component of all cell structures, including muscle structure and function, it takes second place only to oxygen as the most important body component. Unfortunately, most people often overlook this fact.

Since we cannot store or conserve water, it is critical to drink adequate amounts of it every day, especially in hot weather and during physical training. In general, you should consume up to four quarts a day (that's 12 to 16 8-ounce glasses). Ideally you should drink water in intervals throughout the day. Keep a bottle with you at all times. Keep it at your desk so that you can easily take regular drinks. When you exercise you should drink one to two cups of water an hour before you begin and then an additional four to eight ounces every 15 minutes during your workout.

Substances such as alcohol, caffeine, and tobacco increase your body's need for water. Consumed in excess, these substances will harm your body and hinder your performance. Not drinking enough water during physical training or on hot days can result in lack of coordination, irritability, fatigue, muscle cramping, mental confusion—and even more severe problems. Water intake is vital, so stay hydrated!

VITAMINS AND MINERALS

When it comes to supplementing our diets with vitamins people can be passionate. Some people strongly believe that taking a large number of vitamins each day is necessary to maintain or improve their health. However, vitamins are not subject to Food and Drug Administration (FDA) approval, and so manufacturers have wide leeway in marketing these products. You should be careful about taking any vitamins in very large doses (100 times the RDA) as they can be toxic at these levels.

Vitamins and minerals are found in the foods we eat and most nutrition experts agree that the best way to get vitamins is by eating a healthy diet. So, if you eat a healthy diet based on the Pyramid guidelines you probably will get all the vitamins and minerals you need. However, many of us because of poor eating habits, have developed deficiencies—most often in folate, vitamin B6, antioxidants, calcium, and zinc. Taking a daily multivitamin—one that does not exceed the recommended nutrient levels—may be a good way to insure that you are receiving adequate amounts of these nutrients.

Antioxidants are important compounds that preserve and protect your body's cells from the damage of free radicals. Free radicals are oxygen molecules that have split into single electron molecules and can cause tissue damage. Beta carotene, vitamins C and E, and the minerals sulfur and selenium are powerful antioxidants. The following chart provides the US Recommended Daily Allowance for the major vitamins and minerals for adults and children over four. Bear in mind that your age and certain health conditions may call for you to have more or less of a particular vitamin or mineral. Check with your doctor.

VITAMINS

VITAMIN A
FUNCTIONS Prevents night blindness, keeps body tissues healthy, allows for normal bone and teeth growth
BEST FOOD SOURCES Dark, green leafy vegetables, red, orange, or yellow vegetables and fruits, liver, eggs, fish oils, and fortified foods such as milk
REQUIREMENTS 800 to 1000 micrograms retinol equivalents
DEFICIENCY Poor night vision, increased risk of osteomalacia (soft bones), and osteoporosis
TOXICITY Liver damage, bone abnormalities, headaches, double vision, hair loss, vomiting

VITAMIN D
FUNCTIONS Promotes strong bones and teeth
BEST FOOD SOURCES Eggs, cheese, sardines, fortified milk, cereals
REQUIREMENTS 5 to 10 micrograms
DEFICIENCY Increased osteoporosis and osteomalacia risk
TOXICITY Weak muscles and bones, kidney stones, excessive bleeding

VITAMIN E

FUNCTIONS Helps form cell membranes, increases resistance to disease and possibly reduces the risk of certain cancers as well as heart disease

BEST FOOD SOURCES Vegetable oils, seeds, nuts, and wheat germ

REQUIREMENTS 8 to 10 mg alpha-tocopherol equivalents

DEFICIENCY Abnormal nervous system functioning, premature very low birth weight infants

TOXICITY Unknown but very high amounts may interfere with the functioning of other nutrients

VITAMIN K

FUNCTIONS Promotes normal blood clotting

BEST FOOD SOURCES Green leafy vegetables

REQUIREMENTS 55 to 80 micrograms

DEFICIENCY Abnormal blood clotting

TOXICITY None known

VITAMIN C

FUNCTIONS Repairs damaged tissues, promotes wound healing, increases resistance to infection, maintains healthy gums, bones, and teeth

BEST FOOD SOURCES Citrus fruits and juices, tomatoes, potatoes, and raw cabbage

REQUIREMENTS 60 milligrams

DEFICIENCY Scurvy (symptoms may include bleeding, improper wound healing, loose teeth, and swollen gums)

TOXICITY Gastrointestinal pain and diarrhea

VITAMIN B1 (THIAMIN)

FUNCTIONS Carbohydrate metabolism

BEST FOOD SOURCES Whole grains, nuts, peas, beans, pork, enriched breads and cereals

REQUIREMENTS 1 to 1.5 micrograms

DEFICIENCY Weak muscles, nerve damage, fatigue

TOXICITY None known

VITAMIN B2 (RIBOFLAVIN)

FUNCTIONS Energy release and cell repair

BEST FOOD SOURCES Poultry, enriched breads, cereals and grains, as well as green leafy vegetables, organ meats, cheese, milk, and eggs

REQUIREMENTS 1.2 to 1.8 milligrams

DEFICIENCY Sore red tongue, dry flaky skin, cataracts

TOXICITY None known

NIACIN (NICOTINIC ACID)

FUNCTIONS Allows cells to use fuel and oxygen

BEST FOOD SOURCES Meat, fish, poultry, nuts, legumes, enriched cereals and whole grains

REQUIREMENTS 13 to 20 milligrams

DEFICIENCY Pellagra (symptoms may include dermatitis, diarrhea, and dementia)

TOXICITY In very high doses, flushed skin, possible liver damage, high blood sugar, and stomach ulcers

VITAMIN B6 (PYRIDOXINE)

FUNCTIONS Assists in protein and red blood cell formation, helps produce antibodies and hormones.

BEST FOOD SOURCES Meat, chicken, fish, nuts, legumes, and whole grains

REQUIREMENTS 1.5 to 2 milligrams

DEFICIENCY Dermatitis, anemia, convulsions, and nausea

TOXICITY nerve damage

FOLATE (FOLACIN OR FOLIC ACID)

FUNCTIONS Produces DNA and RNA to make cells, helps make red blood cells

BEST FOOD SOURCES Dark green leafy vegetables, orange juice, dried beans, liver, whole grain breads, and cereals

REQUIREMENTS 180 to 200 micrograms

DEFICIENCY Increased risk of spina bifida in offspring, weakness, irritability, sore red tongue, diarrhea, weight loss, anemia

TOXICITY Can mask B12 deficiency, which if untreated, can cause permanent nerve damage

VITAMIN B12 (COBALAMIN)

FUNCTIONS Assists in DNA, RNA and nerve formation, helps make red blood cells, facilitates energy metabolism

BEST FOOD SOURCES Meat, poultry, fish, dairy products, and fortified foods

REQUIREMENTS 2 micrograms

DEFICIENCY Numb hands and feet, fatigue, anemia

TOXICITY None known

BIOTIN

FUNCTIONS Assists in energy production

BEST FOOD SOURCES Eggs, liver, dried beans, nuts, whole grains and cereals

REQUIREMENTS 30 to 100 micrograms

DEFICIENCY Loss of appetite, fatigue, dry skin, heart abnormalities and depression

TOXICITY None known

PANTOTHENIC ACID

FUNCTIONS Assists in energy production

BEST FOOD SOURCES Meat, poultry, fish, whole grains and legumes

REQUIREMENTS 4 to 7 milligrams

DEFICIENCY Numb hands and feet

TOXICITY Diarrhea and water retention

MINERALS

CALCIUM

FUNCTIONS Required for blood clotting, nerve, muscle, and cell membrane functions, builds bone and teeth, promotes enzyme reactions

BEST FOOD SOURCES dairy products, green leafy vegetables, tofu, almonds and legumes

REQUIREMENTS 800 to 1200 milligrams

DEFICIENCY Increases risk for osteoporosis

TOXICITY Kidney stones and damage, constipation

PHOSPHORUS

FUNCTIONS Promotes bone, teeth, DNA and RNA growth, assists in energy production

BEST FOOD SOURCES Meat, poultry, fish, eggs, legumes, nuts and breads

REQUIREMENTS 800 to 1200 milligrams

DEFICIENCY Bone loss, weakness, loss of appetite and pain

TOXICITY Decreases calcium levels in the blood leading to bone loss

MAGNESIUM

FUNCTIONS Component of bones and many enzymes, needed for energy production, muscle contractions, normal nerve and muscle cell functioning

BEST FOOD SOURCES Whole grains, legumes, nuts

REQUIREMENTS 280 to 400 milligrams

DEFICIENCY Muscle tremors, poor coordination, nausea, weakness, convulsions, and poor appetite

TOXICITY Nausea, low blood pressure, heart abnormalities, vomiting

CHROMIUM

FUNCTIONS Allows body to use glucose

BEST FOOD SOURCES Nuts, whole grains, and meat

REQUIREMENTS 50 to 200 micrograms

DEFICIENCY Nerve damage and high blood sugar

TOXICITY None known

COPPER

FUNCTIONS Facilitates energy production, component of enzymes, helps form hemoglobin and connective tissue

BEST FOOD SOURCES Fruits, vegetables, nuts, seeds, legumes, liver

REQUIREMENTS 1.5 to 3 milligrams

DEFICIENCY Anemia

TOXICITY Liver damage, coma, nausea, vomiting, and diarrhea

FLOURIDE

FUNCTIONS Prevents tooth decay, strengthens bones

BEST FOOD SOURCES Sardines, salmon, fluoridated water, and tea

REQUIREMENTS 1.5 to 4 milligrams

DEFICIENCY Tooth decay

TOXICITY Brittle bones, stained or mottled teeth

IODINE

FUNCTIONS Forms hormones that regulate the rate of energy usage

BEST FOOD SOURCES Seafood and table salt

REQUIREMENTS 150 micrograms

DEFICIENCY Enlarged thyroid and weight gain

TOXICITY Enlarged thyroid

IRON

FUNCTIONS Component of hemoglobin that carries oxygen to the cells

BEST FOOD SOURCES Meat, poultry, fish, legumes, green leafy vegetables, dried fruits, and legumes

REQUIREMENTS 10 to 15 milligrams

DEFICIENCY Infections, anemia, and fatigue

TOXICITY Poisonous to children; may lead to hemochromatosis

MANGANESE

FUNCTIONS A component of enzymes involved in energy and protein metabolism

BEST FOOD SOURCES Whole grain products, tea, fruits, and vegetables

REQUIREMENTS 2 to 5 milligrams

DEFICIENCY Rare

TOXICITY Nerve damage

MOLYBDENUM

FUNCTIONS Component of enzymes

BEST FOOD SOURCES Organ meats, milk, legumes, and whole grains

REQUIREMENTS 75 to 250 micrograms

DEFICIENCY Rare

TOXICITY May interfere with copper use

SELENIUM

FUNCTIONS Protects cells from damage, assists with cell growth

BEST FOOD SOURCES Seafood, meats, grains, and seeds

REQUIREMENTS 50 to 70 micrograms

DEFICIENCY May damage the heart

TOXICITY Nerve damage, fatigue, irritability, nausea, vomiting, diarrhea, stomach pain

ZINC

FUNCTIONS Needed for wound healing, growth, reproduction, carbohydrate, protein, and alcohol metabolism, and the making of DNA and RNA

BEST FOOD SOURCES Meat, liver, eggs, dairy, whole grains, legumes, and oysters

REQUIREMENTS 12 to 15 milligrams

DEFICIENCY Loss of senses of taste and smell, loss of appetite, reduced resistance to infection, scaly skin, growth retardation

TOXICITY Interferes with copper absorption and immune functioning, reduces good blood cholesterol (HDL), upsets stomach and may cause nausea and vomiting

SODIUM

FUNCTIONS Regulates fluids, blood pressure, nerve and muscle function

BEST FOOD SOURCES Processed foods and table salt

REQUIREMENTS Minimum of 500 milligrams

DEFICIENCY Muscle cramps, dizziness, nausea, and fatigue

TOXICITY May cause high blood pressure

POTASSIUM

FUNCTIONS Fluid and mineral balance, blood pressure regulation, nerve and muscle function

BEST FOOD SOURCES Fruits, vegetables, poultry, meat, and fish

REQUIREMENTS Minimum of 2000 milligrams
DEFICIENCY Abnormal heartbeat, muscle paralysis, weakness, lethargy
TOXICITY Heart abnormalities

CHLORIDE

FUNCTIONS Component of stomach acid, regulates fluid balance
BEST FOOD SOURCES Table salt
REQUIREMENTS Minimum of 750 milligrams
DEFICIENCY Growth failure, behavioral and learning problems, poor appetite
TOXICITY May cause high blood pressure

READING FOOD LABELS

Learning how to interpret the information on food labels gives you a valuable nutrition tool. The ingredients listed first are the ones present in the highest concentrations by weight. Too often those ingredients are sugar and sodium. Shop for foods that have healthy ingredients front and center.

The serving sizes listed on labels can also be misleading, so you need to examine them carefully. For instance, the label on a small bag of potato chips may list "150 calories per serving," which doesn't sound like much. But read the label more carefully, and you may find that the bag contains *three* servings, not just one. If you eat all of the chips in the bag, you'll have consumed 450 calories.

Finally, it is helpful to know how to convert the nutrients presented on the label in grams to calories to determine how much (energy-wise) of each individual nutrient you would be eating in a serving.

Carbohydrates:	1 gram equals 4 calories
Proteins:	1 gram equals 4 calories
Fats:	1 gram equals 9 calories

When reading labels pay particular attention to the amount of cholesterol and sodium listed. You might be surprised by how many low-fat and low-calorie foods contain high levels of sodium (healthy adults should aim for a total intake

Nutrition Facts

Serving Size 1 oz. (2 cups 28g)
Servings Per Container about 1

Amount Per Serving

Calories 130   Calories from Fat 60

               % Daily Value*

Total Fat 6g	**10**%
Saturated Fat 1g	**5**%
Polyunsaturated Fat 1g	
Monounsaturated Fat 1g	
Cholesterol 0mg	**0**%
Sodium 150mg	**5**%
Total Carbohydrate 17g	**6**%
Dietary Fiber 2g	**8**%
Sugars 1g	
Protein 2g	
Vitamin A	0%
Vitamin C	0%
Calcium	0%
Iron	10%

* Percent Daily Values are based on a 2,000 calorie diet. Your Daily Values may be higher or lower depending on your calorie needs:

	Calories:	2,000	2,500
Total Fat	Less than	65g	80g
Sat Fat	Less than	20g	25g
Cholesterol	Less than	300mg	300mg
Sodium	Less than	2,400mg	2,400mg
Total Carbohydrate		300g	375g
Dietary Fiber		25g	30g

Ingredients: Corn Meal, Canola Oil, Aged Cheddar Cheese, (Milk, Salt, Cheese Cultures, Enzymes), Whey, Buttermilk, Maltodextrin, and Salt.

of no more than 2,400 milligrams per day.) And check to see whether the food contains saturated or hydrogenated oils; if it does, you may want to avoid it because hydrogenated foods contain the unhealthy and potentially harmful trans-fatty acids.

APPENDIX

SELECTED SPECIAL OPS ACRONYMS

AFSOC air force special operations command

BUD/S basic underwater demolition/SEAL training

CA civil affairs

CBT combating terrorism

CD counter drug activities

CP counterproliferation

CSAR combat research and rescue

DA direct action

FID foreign internal defense

HA humanitarian assistance

HD humanitarian demining activities

IO information operations

JFC's joint force commander's

JFSOCC joint force special operations component commander

JSOC joint special operations command

NAVSPECWARCOM naval special warfare command

NSW naval special warfare

PJ parajumper

PSYOP psychological operations

SA security assistance

SB special boat squadrons and units

SEAL sea, air, land

SOF United States special operations forces

SR special reconnaissance

USASOC United States army special operations command

USSOCOM United States special operations command

UW unconventional warfare

WMD weapons of mass destruction

SPECIAL OPS RECRUITING INFORMATION

ARMY SPECIAL FORCES/RANGERS
www.goarmy.com
1-800-USA-ARMY

AIRFORCE SPECIAL OPS
www.airforce.com
1-800-423-USAF

NAVY SEALS
www.sealchallenge.navy.mil
Contact the SEAL Motivators
1-888-USN-SEAL

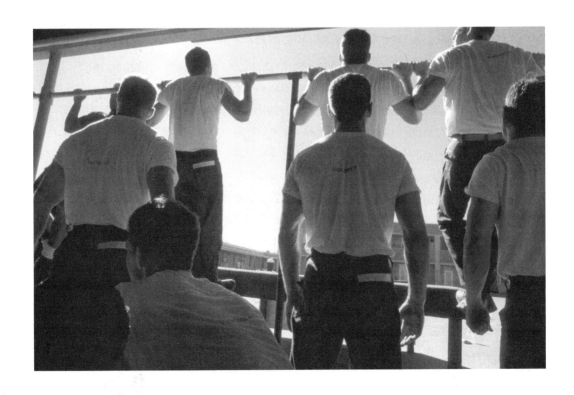

ABOUT THE AUTHORS

Michael Mejia is a certified strength and conditioning specialist and holds a master of science degree in Exercise Science. Michael co-owns Spectrum Conditioning Systems, a sports-specific training center in Port Washington, New York. Throughout his career Michael has worked with a wide variety of athletes. He has served as strength and conditioning consultant to the Saskatoon Blades of the Western Hockey League.

Michael's primary focus these days is on the Young Athlete Development program, which he runs out of his facility, and which is specifically designed to help athletes ages seven to seventeen inprove such qualities as agility, balance, flexibility, speed, and strength.

Michael's work has been featured in such nationally recognized publications as *Muscle & Fitness*, *Oxygen*, *Let's Live*, *Physical* and *Men's Health*. He is a contributing editor and exercise advisor for *Men's Health* magazine.

In addition to his magazine work, Michael's book credits include designing the workout programs for the widely popular *Testosterone Advantage Plan* (Rodale Press, 2000), and *The Home Workout Bible* (Rodale Press, 2002).

Former Navy Lieutenant **Stew Smith** graduated from the United States Naval Academy in 1991 and received orders to Basic Underwater Demolition/SEAL (BUD/S) training (Class 182). Since 1991 he has been developing workouts that prepare future BUD/S students for BUD/S. Those workouts are still in use today by SEAL recruiters. Stew has also authored the books *The BUD/S Warning Order*, *The Complete Guide to Navy SEAL Fitness*, and *Maximum Fitness*.

Fitness has been a part of Stew's life throughout his childhood, high school, Naval Academy, Naval SEAL and present life. His Web site—StewSmith.com—is a window to just about every type of training there is.

ABOUT OUR MODEL

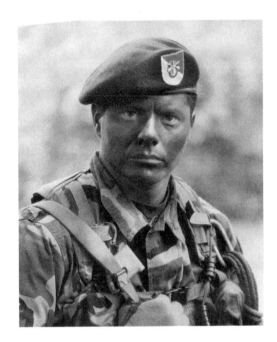

David W. Garcia joined the U.S. Marine Corps in 1977, serving approximately six years. During this period he served as a sergeant, assistant team leader for 2nd Force Recon Co. In 1983 Dave served with the Army's 11th Group Special Forces.

Dave currently serves as a supervisor in the Uniform Patrol Division of the Annapolis City police department in Annapolis, Maryland. His responsibilities have included: Counter-Sniper for the Annapolis Special Emergency Team, detective for Criminal Investigations, and a Field Training officer. In addition, he co-authored the book *Common Sense Self-Defense*.

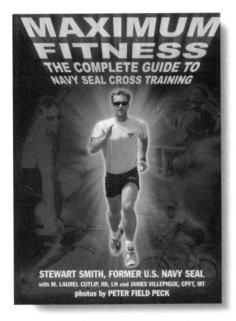

OFFICIAL MILITARY WORKOUT GUIDES!

Add these authorized books to your collection!
Learn the secrets to what keeps America's Armed Forces
in fighting shape!

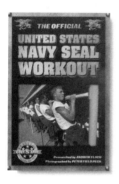
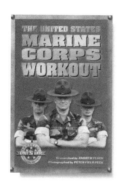

THE OFFICIAL U.S.
NAVY SEAL WORKOUT
ISBN 1-57826-009-4
$14.95

THE OFFICIAL U.S.
MARINE CORPS WORKOUT
ISBN 1-57826-011-6
$14.95

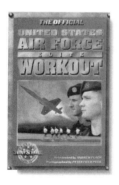
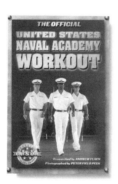

THE OFFICIAL U.S.
AIR FORCE ELITE WORKOUT
ISBN 1-57826-029-9
$14.95

THE OFFICIAL U.S.
NAVAL ACADEMY WORKOUT
ISBN 1-57826-010-8
$14.95

Available wherever books are sold, or direct from the publisher.

Toll-free orders 1-800-906-1234
Order online at www.getfitnow.com

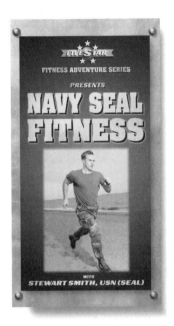

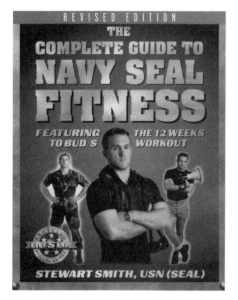